# Velo-Cardio-Facial Syndrome

## Volume I

# Genetic Syndromes and Communication Disorders Series

Robert J. Shprintzen, Ph.D.
*Series Editor*

**Waardenburg Syndrome** by Alice Kahn, Ph.D.

**Educating Children with Velo-Cardio-Facial Syndrome**
by Donna Cutler-Landsman, M.S., Editor

**Medical Genetics: Its Application to Speech, Hearing, and
Craniofacial Disorders** by Nathaniel H. Robin, M.D.

# Velo-Cardio-Facial Syndrome

## Volume I

*A Volume in the*
*Genetics and Communication Disorders Series*

Robert J. Shprintzen, Ph.D.
Karen J. Golding-Kushner, Ph.D.

With contributions from
*Anne Marie Higgins, R.N., F.N.P, M.A. and Abraham Lipton*

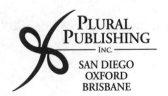

PLURAL
PUBLISHING
INC.

SAN DIEGO
OXFORD
BRISBANE

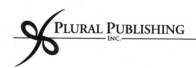

PLURAL PUBLISHING
INC.

5521 Ruffin Road
San Diego, CA 92123

e-mail: info@pluralpublishing.com
Web site: http://www.pluralpublishing.com

49 Bath Street
Abingdon, Oxfordshire OX14 1EA
United Kingdom

**Library of Congress Cataloging-in-Publication Data:**
Shprintzen, Robert J.
  Velo-cardio-facial syndrome / Robert J. Shprintzen and Karen J. Golding-Kushner.
      p. ; cm. – (Genetic syndromes and communication disorders series)
  Includes bibliographical references and index.
  ISBN-13: 978-1-59756-071-9 (alk. paper)
  ISBN-10: 1-59756-071-5 (alk. paper)
  1. Velocardiofacial syndrome.
  [DNLM: 1. DiGeorge Syndrome. QS 675 S5596v 2008] I. Golding-Kushner,
Karen J. II. Title. III. Series.
  RB155.5.S573 2008
  616'.042–dc22
                                                                  2008008002

# Contents

# Preface

*T*his volume is the first of two that are directed towards anyone interested in one of the most common of genetic multiple anomaly disorders in humans, velo-cardio-facial syndrome, or VCFS. Readers may be familiar with the syndrome under a different name, such as DiGeorge syndrome, 22q11 deletion syndrome, conotruncal anomalies face syndrome, Sedlacková syndrome, Cayler syndrome, and Shprintzen syndrome. As discussed in Chapter 1, these different labels all describe the same disorder. We have been involved in the diagnosis, treatment, and study of VCFS for more than 30 years. Our involvement has allowed us to be involved at the professional level with colleagues from all over the world, many of whom came to the study of VCFS somewhat later but with great enthusiasm and a powerful impact. These colleagues have become good friends and generous collaborators. Moreover, we have also been equally involved with thousands of people whose lives have been impacted directly or indirectly by VCFS. Many are people with VCFS, their parents and other relatives, and those who may be caring for people with VCFS in the educational system or health care system. We have both had the privilege of being Executive Director of a wonderful altruistic organization, the Velo-Cardio-Facial Syndrome Educational Foundation, Inc. The people who have participated in this organization, including scientists, clinicians, parents and relatives, people with VCFS, and other interested parties, have instigated the enormous progress in research and clinical care that will be shared in the chapters to follow in this volume. We are eternally grateful to all of them.

This first volume is a more general description of the syndrome and an attempt to integrate scientific knowledge with clinical care, a true exercise in what is commonly called translational research. We have tried to cover as many topics of interest as possible in this book. We feel now, as we did three decades ago, that it is extremely important for everyone to be equipped with a broad base of knowledge covering many different fields to prevent the myopia that often occurs when looking too closely at one specialty only. The transdisciplinary model for providing good care to people with VCFS is critical because the syndrome is so complex.

There are many people we would like to acknowledge, and at the top of our list are our families. Whatever time we have with our families is time that we cherish, and taking some of that away from them is done only because of the importance we assign to these books. We would also like to thank the entire membership of VCFS Educational Foundation, Inc. for what they have given us: knowledge, camaraderie, encouragement, and a very large group of people who function as a second family for both of us. We would also like to thank our friends at Plural Publishing who continue to encourage us and who have added so much to enlighten the community interested in VCFS. Finally, we would like to thank each other, long-standing colleagues and friends. We each feel that our collaboration over these many years exceeds the sum of our parts. "Mutual inspiration" would be an apt description of our many years of parallel and intersecting work.

Robert J. Shprintzen, Ph.D.
Syracuse, NY

Karen J. Golding-Kushner, Ph.D.
East Brunswick, NJ

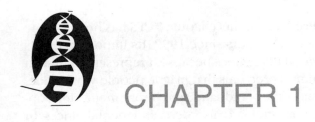

# CHAPTER 1

# The History of VCFS

*V*elo-cardio-facial syndrome (VCFS) is one of the most common multiple anomaly syndromes in humans, probably second in frequency only to Down syndrome (Shprintzen, 2005). VCFS is caused by a deletion of a segment of DNA from chromosome 22 at the q11.2 band that is usually too small to be seen under a microscope (Figure 1–1). Syndromes caused by submicroscopic deletions are known as *microdeletion syndromes*, or *contiguous gene syndromes*.

**Chromosome 22**

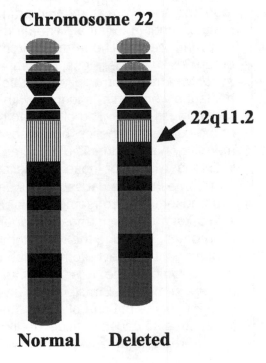

**FIGURE 1–1.** Drawing showing the two copies of chromosome 22 in a person with VCFS. One copy of the chromosome (*right*) has a deletion of DNA from the 22q11.2 locus.

22q11.2

**Normal**   **Deleted**

For reasons that will become clear later in this chapter, VCFS has become one of the most studied human genetic disorders since 1992. Its importance cuts across many medical and behavioral disciplines because it represents a human model for a large number of common problems that plague people worldwide, such as congenital heart disease, speech and language impairment, developmental delay, feeding problems, immunologic disorders, and mental illness. In order to understand the importance of VCFS and its complexity, it is necessary to know something about its history, its cause, and our current level of understanding of this common multiple anomaly disorder. For those reading this text who are not familiar with clinical and molecular genetics, VCFS serves as a launching point for comprehending how a tiny alteration of DNA too small to be seen under a microscope can result in a wide range of disorders, many of which are common in the general population. Congenital heart disease, speech and language impairment, psychiatric disorders, developmental delay, and even autistic spectrum disorder are found in VCFS at rates far higher than might be expected in the general population. It is therefore possible that unlocking the mysteries of how this DNA alteration is responsible for these disorders in VCFS may also help us understand the mechanisms for these problems in people who do not have VCFS.

### What Is a Syndrome?

*Syndrome* is word that has different meanings to different people. The word comes from the Greek roots *sun* (or *syn*), meaning together, and *dromos*, meaning run. The Greek word *sundromos* means "running together." Therefore, a syndrome represents things that run together. The term syndrome is used often to connote groupings of things, signs, or symptoms. The term *Stockholm syndrome* has been applied to a behavioral pattern that develops in hostages who begin to identify with their captors. Irritable bowel syndrome is a grouping of symptoms that result from inflammation of the colon. In genetics, however, syndrome has a more specific meaning. A syndrome is defined as multiple anomalies in a single individual with all of those anomalies having the same cause. Syndromes can be caused by a number of biological events. Chromosome rearrangements that can be seen under a microscope with a karyotype (chromosome analysis) are responsible for many syndromes, including the most common multiple anomaly syndrome in humans, Down syndrome. In the case of Down syndrome, there is typically the presence of an entire extra chromosome (chromosome 21). Smaller DNA arrangements that cannot be seen on a karyotype but can often be detected with molecular genetics tests can also cause multiple anomaly syndromes. Most of these smaller rearrangements happen within a single gene and are therefore called single gene disorders. Single gene disorders probably account for the majority of human genetic disease and may occur as new spontaneous mutations in DNA or can be inherited. Another type of submicroscopic DNA rearrangement is known as a microdeletion (also called a contiguous gene syndrome) where there is a deletion of DNA that spans more than one gene. VCFS is a microdeletion syndrome and it is presumed that all of the anomalies are caused by the deletion of a segment of DNA from chromosome 22. Another possible cause of syndromes is maternal exposure to teratogens. Teratogens include drugs, environmental contaminants, viruses, and hyperthermia.

### Are All Multiple Anomaly Disorders Syndromes?

There are some groupings of symptoms that do not meet the criteria for definition as syndromes. These are called sequences. A sequence is defined as multiple anomalies in a single individual with some or all of those anomalies caused secondarily by the presence of another anomaly that has interfered with the normal process of morphogenesis. In other words, an abnormal embryonic developmental process results in the presence of an anomaly. Once that anomaly is present, it interrupts the normal development of the embryo by interfering with the development of tissues and structures adjacent to it. This seems complicated, but it can be understood within the context of Robin sequence, a grouping of symptoms that had been previously and incorrectly labeled as Pierre Robin syndrome. Now known as Robin sequence, the symptom complex includes the association of a small or retruded lower jaw (micrognathia or retrognathia), a wide U-shaped cleft of the secondary palate, and upper airway obstruction presumed to be caused by glossoptosis (the tongue dropping postero-inferiorly into the airway). In the case of Robin sequence, the palatal cleft and upper airway obstruction (glossoptosis) are actually secondary findings that have only occurred because of the presence of the micrognathia or retrognathia. The sequence occurs as follows. During embryogenesis, at approximately 9 to 11 weeks' development, the lower jaw is typically quite small and the oral cavity is also very small. The tongue sits flush against the skull base (Figure 1–2) until there is a rapid burst of mandibular growth that enlarges the oral cavity so that the tongue can descend into the floor of the oral cavity (Figure 1–2). As the tongue drops from between the palatal shelves, they are free to swing into a horizontal position and grow towards the midline where they fuse, creating an intact palate (Figure 1–2). If the mandible did not grow resulting in enlargement of the oral cavity, the tongue would remain between the palatal shelves, therefore preventing them from fusing. As the cranium continues to expand laterally and the tongue remains against the skull base, the palatal shelves will eventually lose the potential to grow medially and fuse. This fusion failure results in a U-shaped cleft of the secondary palate consistent with the contour of the tongue. At birth, the small mandible will cause the tongue to be retropositioned in the airway leading to glossoptosis and airway obstruction. This sequence of events is caused by the presence of a single anomaly, a small or retruded mandible. However, small or retruded mandibles have many possible causes. Many genetic syndromes have micrognathia or retrognathia (or both) as clinical features, including VCFS, Stickler syndrome, and Treacher Collins syndrome, among others. Larger chromosome rearrangements may also have mandibular anomalies as features, including Turner syndrome (45×) and trisomy 13. Mandibular anomalies can also be caused by exposure to teratogens, such as alcohol and hydantoins, and by fetal positioning abnormalities, such as a breech presentation and intrauterine crowding. The concept of a sequence is important to mention in the context of VCFS because single anomalies that are part of its phenotype trigger a number of secondary sequences, including Robin sequence, DiGeorge sequence, and holoprosencephaly sequence. It is well known that individual features of many syndromes can trigger developmental sequences. It is therefore possible to be diagnosed with both a syndrome and a sequence.

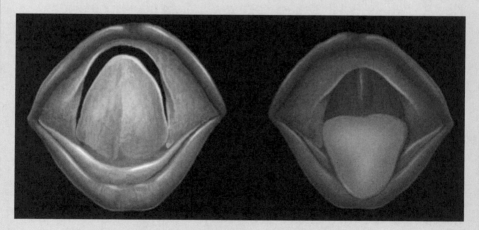

**FIGURE 1–2.** The mechanism for the presence of cleft palate in Robin sequence showing the intervention of the tongue between the palatal shelves (*left*) preventing them from fusing and causing a U-shaped cleft palate after the tongue descends in the oral cavity (*right*).

# THE HISTORY OF VCFS

The delineation of genetically caused syndromes is not an instant process. Rarely is it ever confined to one "Eureka" moment, and it is also rarely confined to one person shouting "Eureka." Even Down syndrome, which has become so inexorably identified with John Langdon Haydon Down who described it in 1866, was described more than 20 years earlier by Séguin (1846) in the French literature, and probably even earlier by others. Velo-cardio-facial syndrome is no different.

The term velo-cardio-facial syndrome, often shortened to VCFS for convenience, was coined in a 1978 paper that reported 12 cases of individuals with a similar pattern of malformations and developmental problems (Shprintzen et al., 1978). A dozen anomalies were reported as consistent features that included palate anomalies (hence the term *velo* for velum, the Latin word for soft palate), heart malformations (*cardio*), and a characteristic facial appearance (*facial*). Also included in the list of features were learning disabilities, inguinal hernia, chronic middle ear disease, abundant scalp hair, minor ear anomalies, and slender and tapered digits. Included among the reported cases were one patient with Robin sequence and one familial case with an affected mother and her daughter. Autosomal dominant inheritance was suspected, although it could not be confirmed without a male-to-male transmission that would rule out X-linked inheritance. The palate anomalies were highly variable, ranging from overt cleft palate (including the wide U-shaped cleft in the single Robin sequence case) to occult submucous cleft palate. The series of cases was reported specifically to delineate a new genetic syndrome. However, the 1978 report was not the first to describe cases of the syndrome, and an earlier report of a single family was actually the first publication to delineate the disorder as a specific syndrome.

The first published report that included cases with VCFS was probably that of Sedláčková in 1955 with a follow-up report in 1967. Sedláčková's 1955 paper was a description of the symptom of hypernasal speech in a small series of cases that was hypothesized to be related to congenital shortening of the velum. In 1967, Sedláčková further described lack of facial animation and possible innervation problems associated with this condition. In reviewing photographs and clinical information from her early papers, it is evident that at least some of the cases, but probably not all, described by Sedláčková had VCFS. Sedláčková was not describing this condition as a specific genetic syndrome, but rather as an explanation for the speech problems presented by these cases. The articles did not draw much attention at the time because the first paper was published in a Czechoslovakian medical journal. At the time, Czechoslovakia was still behind the Iron Curtain, a part of the Soviet bloc. There was very little scientific interaction between the medical communities in the United States and Western Europe and their fellow scientists in the communist world of Eastern Europe. Sedláčková's 1967 paper was published in a speech and voice journal, *Folia Phoniatrica*. Although an international journal, *Folia Phoniatrica* was read primarily by specialists in speech and voice disorders and as a result did not receive wide attention from other medical specialists. In any event, at the time, people interested in clinical genetics would probably not have been aware of articles in that journal, especially without the advantage of computer databases like PubMed and Medline that are available today. In addition, clinical genetics was a very limited field in 1955 and 1967. Very few clinicians studied human genetics or dysmorphology at the time. It was not until the late 1970s that dysmorphology became a more expansive field of study. Genetics did not become a true medical specialty with board certification until 1991 and it is not likely that disorders described prior to that time, especially in journals not specifically associated with genetic disorders, would receive much attention.

In 1968, Angelo DiGeorge, a pediatric endocrinologist at St. Christopher's Hospital in Philadelphia, described an association of symptoms in newborns with congenital heart disease that included absence of the thymus gland, hypoparathyroidism, and resulting hypocalcemia with severe immune deficiency (DiGeorge, 1968) in the birth defects literature. At that time, infants with this symptom complex did not survive the neonatal period, so it was unlikely that there would have been a chance to observe the condition over time to fully delineate its clinical phenotype. However, later that year, Roberto Kretschmer, a pediatric endocrinologist from Mexico, reported a child with "DiGeorge's syndrome" in *The New England Journal of Medicine*. Photographs of that child clearly demonstrate a facial appearance consistent with VCFS. The articles of DiGeorge and Kretschmer approached these cases as endocrine and immune disorders related to abnormal development of the 3rd and 4th branchial pouches, and no familial cases were presented. It is now known that the association of athymia, hypoparathyroidism, hypocalcemia, and congenital heart disease is a sequence, not a syndrome. DiGeorge sequence occurs in association with a number of multiple anomaly disorders including del(10p), del(17p), caudal regression syndrome, Zellweger syndrome, peroxisomal disorders (Robin and Shprintzen, 2005), fetal alcohol syndrome, CHARGE, Down syndrome, Kabuki syndrome (Niikawa–Kuroki syndrome), de Lange syndrome (Shprintzen, 2005), and most commonly with VCFS.

Also in 1968, the first article appeared that delineated this condition as a distinct genetic syndrome written by William Strong, a pediatric cardiologist at the Medical College of Georgia. Strong described a family of a mother and three children who clearly had VCFS. His description included the findings of right-sided aortic arch and mental retardation, but he did not mention speech impairment. In 1981, our research group was about to publish our third paper on VCFS when a resident at our hospital, Robert W. Marion, M.D. (currently Professor of Pediatrics and Obstetrics and Gynecology at the Albert Einstein College of Medicine, Director of the Center for Congenital Disorders at Montefiore Medical Center in the Bronx, and Director, Children's Evaluation and Rehabilitation Center) found the article by Strong. We called Dr. Strong and in an effort to determine if he was describing the same syndrome, asked him if his patients had abnormal speech. His answer was written down and he kindly allowed us to acknowledge it in our paper. He said, "Funny you should ask that. None of them had cleft palate, but they all sounded like they did." It is likely that Strong's patients had occult submucous cleft palate (Croft, Shprintzen, Daniller, & Lewin, 1978; Kaplan, 1975; Lewin, Croft, & Shprintzen, 1980; Shprintzen, 1979).

Although Strong's article was an excellent description of VCFS based on the understanding of clinical genetics at the time, syndromes described in single families did not receive substantial attention in a field that was still in its infancy. However, Strong is not given nearly enough credit for his important role in delineating a previously unrecognized syndrome of genetic causation and his article provided a sound basis for suspecting autosomal dominant transmission.

In 1976, Kinouchi et al. published a series of cases with conotruncal heart anomalies and a characteristic facial appearance. The large majority of these cases had VCFS and the disorder came to be known as conotruncal anomalies face syndrome (CAFS) in Japan. As with Sedláčková's earlier publication, the Kinouchi article received little attention because it was published

---

### What Is Occult Submucous Cleft Palate?

Occult submucous cleft palate is a term that was coined by Kaplan in 1975. Kaplan, a plastic surgeon at Stanford, reported four patients who were referred for pharyngeal flap surgery secondary to the complaint of hypernasal speech. On oral examination, the palate was found to be intact with no evidence of bifurcation of the uvula or notching of the hard palate. When the patients were taken to surgery, the palate was explored surgically, and the orientation of the muscle fibers was abnormal consistent with that typically seen in submucous cleft palate. Of interest, of the four cases in Kaplan's report, it is clear from facial photographs that three of them had VCFS. Kaplan concluded that the only way that this anomaly could be detected was by surgical dissection. However, several years later, Croft et al. (1978), Shprintzen (1979), and Lewin et al. (1980) described the endoscopic findings associated with occult submucous cleft palate and indicated that endoscopic view of the nasal surface of the velum can detect the occult submucous cleft. The hallmark of this anomaly is absence of the musculus uvulae or a concavity of the nasal surface of the velum. This anomaly will be described in further detail in Chapter 2. Video 1–1 on the DVD demonstrates an occult submucous cleft in comparison to a normal appearing palate.

in a Japanese language journal. Non-English language journals were more easily overlooked in the years that preceded electronic publication databases such as OVID, Medline, and PubMed. Also, in the years prior to on-line access to full text journal articles, access to foreign language journals in American medical libraries was limited.

At the time our article was published in 1978, clinical genetics was a burgeoning field with many publications beginning to appear in a large number of medical and dental journals. A small number of journals were almost exclusively devoted to the report of new syndromes. Prior to this time, the study of multiple anomaly syndromes was referred to as *teratology*. The formal definition of teratology is the branch of biology and medical science that studies the development of malformations or deviations from normal in organisms. The root of this term, *teratos*, translates as *monster* in Greek. The term teratology or teratologist is not used much any longer. In part, it is because this is an older lexicon that preceded the development of human genetics as a prominent field in medicine. However, it is also true that the root, *teratos*, meaning monster, is pejorative, and scientists and clinicians should be sensitive to the offense created by the use of pejorative terms. Perhaps worse has been the common use of the term *funny looking kid* (often abbreviated to FLK) that is even more denigrating to people who have differences from the norm. Therefore, in the 1970s, clinicians and scientists began to refer to the study of birth defects as *dysmorphology* or *syndromology*. Thousands of new syndromes were delineated in the 1970s and 1980s and it was in this climate that our article describing VCFS first appeared in 1978.

The term syndromology is not really in use any longer, and even dysmorphology seems dated, although many clinicians still use it. With the enormous surge in research and expansion of knowledge in human genetics since the early 1990s, medical genetics became a board certified specialty in 1991. Genetic counselors also have a board certification process. Today, those clinicians who were previously called dysmorphologists or syndromologists are now called clinical geneticists, and the majority of them are coming from the field of pediatrics. The development of techniques to analyze DNA and to match those analyses to clinical findings led to more efficient and accurate diagnoses of genetic diseases with concomitant understanding of the biological mechanisms that cause them. Therefore, today the diagnostic process has become far more scientific and less dependent on judgment and interpretation. With many genetic mutations identified and many thousands of multiple anomaly syndromes described, there are fewer discoveries of new disorders today than 20 years ago. The result is that familiar syndromes are recognized earlier and more frequently. This is actually easy to document. We saw approximately 70 new patients with VCFS in 1985 and also in 2006. In 1985, all but one of the patients we saw were new diagnoses of the syndrome at their first visit. All had been referred for problems of speech, feeding, cleft palate, or other craniofacial manifestations. In 2006, all but two of the patients came in with the diagnosis of VCFS already established. Approximately 75% of those cases were detected because of the presence of congenital heart disease with many cases of tetralogy of Fallot, interrupted aortic arch, and truncus arteriosus among the sample. The balance of the referrals was related to speech, feeding, and developmental disorders and two cases to psychiatric manifestations as diagnostic clues. This shift in the diagnostic recognition of VCFS began in 1992 with two major events that occurred nearly simultaneously.

## TWO MAJOR EVENTS IN 1992

In 1991, we received a number of telephone calls from patients with VCFS we had seen as early as 1974 as young children who had been referred initially for velopharyngeal insufficiency. Their speech problems had been treated successfully and they had been discharged from active follow-up after several years. The telephone calls were questions, asking if psychiatric illness could possibly be a part of the phenotypic spectrum of VCFS. These patients had been diagnosed by a number of community psychiatrists to have schizophrenia and other psychoses. These calls brought to mind two patients I had seen in my earliest series of cases, one of whom had been diagnosed with childhood schizophrenia at 14 years, and an adult male, age 61, who had been a long-term resident of a psychiatric institute with the diagnosis of chronic schizophrenia. Although these two cases both had significant psychiatric illness, the large percentage of patients being followed at the time were school-age children who had not yet developed significant signs of mental illness. Current data suggest that nearly one third of individuals with VCFS may develop significant psychiatric illness and that the average age of onset is in late adolescence or early adult life. Therefore, the cases being followed at the time were unlikely to be demonstrating psychosis. However, in 1992, many of the patients originally described in 1978 were young adults and the recognition of their mental illness was age sensitive (Shprintzen, Goldberg, Golding-Kushner, & Marion, 1992). Of the original 12 subjects described in 1978, 5 have developed severe mental illness. Because one of the cases described in 1978 died in early childhood, this means that nearly half of this small sample went on to develop psychosis or severe psychiatric disease. Even if the most conservative estimates of the frequency of mental illness in VCFS are true, the frequency of psychosis in VCFS is approximately 25 times greater than that in the general population.

In May of the same year, the genetic cause of VCFS was identified. The early reports of Strong (1968), Shprintzen et al. (1978, 1981), Williams et al. (1985), and Meinecke et al. (1986) described autosomal dominant transmission of VCFS. Microdeletion syndromes (originally referred to as contiguous gene syndromes) were not known as specific diagnostic entities until 1986 and because deletions that occur on an autosome are expressed as autosomal dominant disorders, the original assumption was that they represented single gene mutations. It was not until 1992 that it was recognized that VCFS was a microdeletion syndrome encompassing multiple genes. In 1991, our research group made contact with Dr. Peter Scambler in London. Dr. Scambler was studying chromosome 22 and was particularly interested in what many people referred to as DiGeorge syndrome. The interest in children with DiGeorge syndrome was the presence of congenital heart disease, hypoparathyroidism, and immune disorders. In 1981, de la Chapelle et al. had reported a family with an unusual unbalanced translocation that resulted in the loss of an interstitial segment of chromosome 22 that they thought involved the q11 band. At that time, it was not known that the conditions previously labeled as "DiGeorge" and "velo-cardio-facial syndrome" actually represented the same condition, but we had reported earlier that some individuals with VCFS had features of DiGeorge (hypocalcemia and hypoparathyroidism) as a secondary developmental sequence (Goldberg, Marion, Borderon, Wiznia, & Shprintzen, 1985). Dr. Scambler's interests in the 22q11 region were focused on DiGeorge while our research was focused on VCFS. After reviewing photos and clinical records of some of Dr. Scambler's cases, it became clear that we were all interested in the same disorder. In order to determine if VCFS was caused by the same deletion from chromosome 22, with or without the presence of the findings consistent with DiGeorge sequence, half of the samples given to Dr. Scambler had no history of heart anomalies, immune disorders, or hypocalcemia. The other half had heart anomalies and a variety of endocrine and immune problems. All of the cases were found to have the deletion and the results published in *The Lancet* (Scambler et al., 1992). Later that year, we provided a similar series of DNA samples to another laboratory performing similar research at the Children's Hospital of Philadelphia that were pooled with a number of their own cases. The results were the same and were published 4 months later in the *American Journal of Medical Genetics* (Driscoll et al., 1992). These studies confirmed a cause for VCFS, but also confirmed that clinicians had assigned a number of different names to the same condition. The deletions observed in patients who had been labeled as VCFS were exactly the same as the deletions in those diagnosed with DiGeorge syndrome in the United States and conotruncal anomalies face syndrome in Japan. Studies in the years that followed also demonstrated that patients who had been identified as having Cayler syndrome and Sedláčková syndrome shared the same deletion (Fokstuen et al., 2001; Giannotti, Digilio, Marino, Mingarelli, & Dallapiccola, 1994).

## The Implications

The implications of this 1992 concurrence of findings in VCFS spurred an enormous amount of excitement in the research community and changed the direction of the study of VCFS. The coordinated findings of the high frequency of mental illness in VCFS and a consistent deletion from chromosome

22 were the first hard evidence of a possible genetic cause of mental illness. Therefore, researchers embarked on two paths in an attempt to bring these two findings together. The full impact of the finding cannot be understated. For years, scientists have argued back and forth about the so-called "nature versus nurture" issue. When it comes to behavior, how much is related to our individual genome? The argument has political, legal, moral, ethical, and even religious overtones and has caused more than a few major conflicts that have been played out in the press and in the courts. Perhaps it is time to put the nature versus nurture argument behind us and frame it as a nature *and* nurture issue. It is well known that the genome interacts with the environment in many ways, and even mutations that cause maladaptive traits may not cause problems without a specific environmental interaction. For example, albinism is caused by a number of different genetic mutations. Most forms of albinism result in depigmentation of the skin, hair, irises, and retinas. The major problems associated with this depigmentation are susceptibility to sunburn and skin cancers resulting from repeated sun exposure, and the potential for visual impairment with nystagmus, although this is also variable. People with albinism function better visually in low light situations, and will not get sunburn and resulting skin cancers if they are not exposed to too much direct sunlight. Therefore, people with albinism who live in darkened environments will feel little impact from the disease. Although this is a bit of an oversimplification, the concept is similar for susceptibility to other genetically caused diseases, including metabolic disorders and certain cancers. It may be postulated that behavioral problems, including speech and language disorders, represent a combination of genomic predisposition combined with environmental triggers.

## COMMUNICATION DISORDERS AND VCFS

In the early years of syndromology and clinical genetics, there was a strong emphasis on physical (i.e., structural) anomalies. In part, this emphasis was on the obvious: anomalies that could be seen, characterized, and measured for easy description. Because so few syndromes had been delineated compared to the current number, identifying combinations of obvious anomalies like abnormal facial or unusual limb malformations was a much easier process. Very few behavioral problems were discussed as features of syndromes at the time with the exception of cognitive impairment and its consequences. Nearly all of the scientists and clinicians who engaged in syndrome delineation at the time were from fields of physical science in medicine and dentistry that focused on structure. Few behavioral scientists participated in the process 30 years ago. Psychiatrists and other behavioral clinicians began to join the process in the 1990s when it became obvious that a significant percentage of mental illness had a genetic basis. Neuropsychologists and developmental pediatricians also became important participants in the study of genetic disorders more recently. However, those in the field of communication science have been slow to engage in the study of multiple anomaly syndromes and to participate in how the genome can contribute to speech, language, and hearing disorders.

Multiple anomaly syndromes are often delineated because of one or more key striking features that are accompanied by a recognizable pattern. The more unusual the key finding is, the easier it is to narrow in on a possible diagnosis. For example, in EEC syndrome (ectrodactyly, ectodermal dysplasia, and clefting), the ectrodactyly (a severe limb malformation involving missing digits and clefting of the hand) is a rare finding that is shared by very few genetic syndromes, so when it is seen, EEC enters the differential diagnosis immediately. When ectodermal dysplasia is also present, the diagnosis is all but certain. It is also true that the delineation of many syndromes is dependent on recognition by specialists who are observant of congenital malformations. With the exception of potentially severe congenital heart problems, velo-cardio-facial syndrome does not typically have severe or striking structural malformations as prominent characteristics. Velo-cardio-facial syndrome was recognized in large part because of a consistent communication impairment that was distinctive and nearly syndrome specific. Speech disorders are behavioral impairments and as such had not typically been considered to be congenital anomalies in the same vein as heart and limb malformations. There was also generally a presumption that speech disorders such as language and articulation impairments were learned at least in large part. More recently, however, direct genetic links to speech disorders have been identified (Fisher, Vargha-Khadem, Watkins, Monaco, & Pembrey, 1998). Obviously, the development of speech is a complex process that involves the interaction of the ability to take thoughts and mental processes and represent them symbolically with spoken sounds. The physical component of making speech sounds involves the respiratory system, oral structures, coordination supplied by the brain and peripheral nerves, and muscular movements that require coordination so that the sounds made are consistent with the extant expressive language. Therefore, genetic mutations could affect one or more of these components that would secondarily result in disorders of speech. Consistency of the communicative impairment would depend on the consistency of expression of that particular genetic trait. In VCFS, there is a common, although not perfectly consistent, speech and language phenotype that has multiple contributors to its expression.

The initial association of symptoms that called attention to VCFS was severe hypernasality and congenital heart disease. Although the combination of hypernasality and heart anomalies can occur in a number of other syndromes (fetal alcohol syndrome, Down syndrome, Kabuki syndrome, CHARGE syndrome, Opitz syndrome, Turner syndrome, and Noonan syndrome, to name a few), the pattern of hypernasality with compensatory articulation substitutions in the absence of apparent cleft palate in VCFS was distinctive (this will be described in detail in Chapter 2). Why was this association seen so frequently within a relatively short period of time in a single center? Is there something inherent in congenital heart disease that would contribute to abnormal speech? Is there a strong association between congenital heart anomalies and cleft palate? The reason that VCFS was recognized as a specific syndrome was because the hypernasality was regarded as an anomaly and not as an incidental finding.

## The Significance of Two Anomalies Occurring Together

Why would there be suspicion that a child (or adult, for that matter) has a syndrome if the child demonstrates two different problems? In the case of hypernasal speech associated with cleft palate or submucous cleft palate (common findings in VCFS), and congenital heart anomalies, the clinician is faced with two common problems. It is tempting to believe that it is coincidental if two common problems could frequently coexist in the same child. Shprintzen (1997) previously discussed that the probability of this type of association would be rare. Actually, the association should be far rarer than previously estimated. The frequency of congenital heart disease is approximately 1:400 births. The frequency of cleft palate including submucous cleft palate is not really known because submucous cleft palate is not often detected at birth and may only become noticed when hypernasal speech is present. Shprintzen (1997) used the common estimate of 1:750 people born with cleft palate, with or without cleft lip. The probability of congenital heart disease and clefting (of all types) occurring together strictly by chance would be 1:750 × 400, or 1:300,000. Cleft lip is uncommon in VCFS, with most cases having cleft palate and most of those being submucous or occult submucous clefts. However, Shprintzen et al. (1985) found that the large majority of individuals with submucous cleft palate have normal speech. In a sample ascertained from a general pediatric practice, less than 5% of individuals with submucous cleft palate were found to have hypernasal speech (Shprintzen, Schwartz, Daniller, & Hoch, 1985). It is also known that the majority of people, probably more than 80%, with repaired clefts of the palate do not have hypernasal speech after surgery. Therefore, the frequency of hypernasality in the cleft population is significantly lower than the frequency of clefting. If the frequency of clefting is 1:750, but only a fraction of those cases were hypernasal, then the frequency of hypernasal speech secondary to palate anomalies would be lower. Even if one third of individuals with palate anomalies were hypernasal, that would reduce the frequency of hypernasal speech in children to approximately 1:2250 (i.e., three times 750). The probability of these two problems occurring together in the same child by chance would be the same as having two barrels filled with ping-pong balls, one with 2250 and the other with 400 with one ball in each barrel painted red. The probability of the two anomalies, heart and hypernasality, occurring together by chance would be the probability that after the two barrels are shaken and the balls mixed, someone would stick one hand in one barrel and the other hand in the other barrel and pick out the two red ping-pong balls. That probability is $1:400 \times 2250$, or $1:900,000$. Because a dozen patients with this same pattern of anomalies were seen in a short period of time in a single center in one location in the United States at a time when there were slightly more than 3,000,000 births per year (meaning one would expect three or four births per year with this combination), there must be some other explanation for this frequent occurrence. VCFS has a population prevalence of $1:2000$ (Shprintzen, 2005; Robin and Shprintzen, 2005).

It is interesting to note that several studies have found that a high percentage of patients referred to cleft palate/craniofacial centers have VCFS. Shprintzen et al. (1985) reported that 8.1% of patients with clefts of the secondary palate at their cleft palate center had VCFS. This sample included individuals with submucous cleft palate or occult submucous cleft palate (Croft et al., 1978; Kaplan, 1975; Lewin et al., 1980; Shprintzen, 1979). Shprintzen et al. (1985) noted that the majority of VCFS cases had submucous and occult submucous clefts of the palate. Lipson et al. (1991) found that approximately 5% of the patients at their cleft palate center in Sydney, Australia, had VCFS. They did not differentiate between clefts of the secondary palate alone and clefts of the lip and palate. One patient in the sample of 38 cases reported by Lipson et al. had a cleft lip. Our own clinical experience is that VCFS is the most common cause of occult submucous cleft palate.

## The Implications for Speech Pathologists, Surgeons, and Other Craniofacial Specialists

Although VCFS is being recognized much more frequently today, the majority of diagnoses are being made because of the presence of conotruncal heart anomalies. The frequency of heart anomalies and velopharyngeal insufficiency (VPI) in VCFS is approximately the same (approximately 70% of cases), but they do not perfectly overlap. Many of the cases who do not have heart anomalies are detected in early childhood because of hypernasality and other speech impairments, but these detections may be relatively late when compared to the age of diagnosis for those with congenital heart disease, such as 3, 4, or 5 years of age. Common among infants and toddlers with VCFS are early feeding problems, nasal regurgitation (usually mistakenly called "nasal reflux"), delayed onset of speech, and mild language delay. One or more of these findings occur in nearly all children with VCFS. It seems the diagnosis is being missed in infants and toddlers, many of whom are being treated in hospital-based feeding programs. A more detailed discussion of the communication phenotypes is found in Chapter 2.

## WHAT DO I CALL IT?

The issue of nosology (the classification of diseases) is impacted by how people name conditions. In the case of VCFS, the confusion over terminology has created a great deal of misunderstanding that persists in many locations.

Earlier in this chapter, the contributions of Sedláčková, DiGeorge, Cayler, and Japanese authors were discussed. Because all of these reports were published in different journals and from different perspectives, each became named with a specific eponym (DiGeorge, Cayler, Sedláčková, Shprintzen) or symptomatic descriptor (conotruncal anomalies face syndrome, velo-cardio-facial syndrome) or primary cause (22q11 deletion syndrome). The acronym CATCH 22 was also suggested (cardiac abnormality/abnormal facies, T-cell deficit due to thymic hypoplasia, cleft palate, hypocalcemia caused by a deletion from chromosome 22) by Wilson et al. (1993). CATCH 22 has been rejected because it is an attempt at humor at the expense of affected individuals. CATCH 22 is the title of a black humor novel by Joseph Heller and is a term reserved for a no-win situation, or an impossible circumstance with no solution (Robin & Shprintzen, 2005). Inside jokes in health care should be rejected without a moment's hesitation.

Because the syndrome has several labels that have been applied in a variety of literature sources and in clinical practice, some clinicians and researchers have mistakenly concluded that each label represents a separate and specific syndrome, each caused by the same deletion from chromosome 22 (Robin & Shprintzen, 2005). It has been emphasized that VCFS is a syndrome with highly variable clinical expression, as one might expect in a disorder caused by a deletion of a large segment of DNA. Even single gene mutations can result in significantly variable clinical expression, but when more genes are in play, the potential for increased variability is increased. Experienced clinicians recognize that all individuals with the same syndrome are not "cookie cutter" consistent.

Another problem is that several authors have claimed that a number of syndromes that have phenotypic overlap with VCFS are also caused by the same 22q11.2 deletion. Both Fryburg et al. (1996) and McDonald-McGinn et al. (1996) reported that Opitz syndrome (also known as Opitz G/BBB syndrome) is caused by the same deletion. The reason for this conclusion is that some people with VCFS have orbital hypertelorism (wide-spaced eyes), swallowing problems, and other anomalies consistent with Opitz syndrome such as cleft palate and hypospadias. Opitz syndrome as originally described has been confirmed to be X-linked; another disorder similar to Opitz syndrome was mapped to chromosome 22, but none of the cases linked to chromosome 22 were caused by a deletion. Reviewing Fryburg's case, there is nothing in the photos or the clinical report that is inconsistent with VCFS, but key features of Opitz syndrome are not present. It is clear that an incorrect assignment of diagnostic label has created considerable nosologic confusion by misclassification of the disease.

As discussed by Robin and Shprintzen (2005), if an individual has a deletion from chromosome 22 at the q11.2 band, then he or she has VCFS (or 22q11 deletion syndrome or whatever other label you choose), and if there is no deletion, then the individual does not have the syndrome. It is also true that any diagnostic label that involves the same 22q11.2 deletion represents exactly the same disorder regardless of the name applied. This is no trivial matter in relation to managing the syndrome. Specific conditions may require syndrome-specific management. For example, the case reported by Fryburg et al. (1996) as having Opitz syndrome would have been explored for a laryngotracheal cleft, perhaps by bronchoscopy under anesthesia. Laryngotracheal clefts are not clinical features in VCFS. Conversely, if this patient requires pharyngeal surgery, such as a pharyngeal flap, it would be very important to know if the diagnosis is VCFS. Anomalies of the internal carotid arteries are common in VCFS and may present as major surgical risks if not identified by appropriate angiographic diagnostic procedures (Mitnick, Bello, Golding-Kushner, Argamaso, & Shprintzen, 1996; Tatum, Chang, Havkin, & Shprintzen, 2002). Internal carotid anomalies have not been identified in Opitz syndrome (or any other syndrome for that matter) and therefore would not be routinely assessed if pharyngeal surgery were necessary, therefore exposing the patient to potentially dangerous surgical complications.

It would certainly be helpful if there were not a variety of names being applied to the same condition. So why the application of so many different names? As implied earlier, it is likely that in some cases the problem is purely geographic. It is understandable that from a position of national pride or perception, the first person to describe the disorder should be honored, and the use of Sedláčková syndrome in Eastern Europe, or conotruncal anomalies face syndrome in Japan, DiGeorge syndrome in Philadelphia, or Shprintzen syndrome in Syracuse and New York might be expected. Some authors have advocated for the use of 22q11.2 deletion syndrome. This seems curious for a microdeletion syndrome. Chromosomal deletion syndromes (those involving microscopically detectable chromosome rearrangements) are often labeled in this manner, although not always. For example, Wolf-Hirschhorn syndrome is most typically known by its eponym, not 4p16 deletion syndrome, and the same is true for cri-du-chat syndrome (an unfortunate descriptor from the sound of the baby's cry being catlike), which is not typically referred to as 5p15 deletion syndrome. Microdeletion syndromes like VCFS are essentially never identified by their deletion site. Williams syndrome has never been known as 7q11 deletion syndrome although, like VCFS, there is no other cause of Williams syndrome, and everyone who has a deletion at 7q11.23 has Williams syndrome. It is for this reason that we advocate calling the disorder VCFS, which is descriptive, geographically nonspecific, free of eponyms, and much easier to write and say than 22q11.2 deletion syndrome.

Diagnostic accuracy leads to treatment accuracy. Understanding the nature of VCFS is dependent on making sure that individuals with the syndrome who are being studied, whether in a clinical or research model, all have the same disorder. Variable expression of genetic disorders is a well-known phenomenon. Seeing phenotypic differences between individuals who have the same syndrome should not lead scientists to split apart the disorder with different names for the various expressions. Rather, we need to understand how these differences come about based on the genomic nature of the deletion, modifying genes that may interact with 22q11.2, and how the environment and epigenetic factors influence the expression.

## VIDEO IN THIS CHAPTER

**Video 1–1:** Nasopharyngoscopy of a normal palate showing a promi-nent midline convexity representing the muscle mass of the musculus uvulae, followed by an endoscopic view of the nasal surface of the palate in a child with VCFS, showing a midline concavity indicating absence of the musculus uvulae.

## REFERENCES

Budarf, M. L., Konkle, B. A., Ludlow, L. B., Michaud, D., Li, M., Yamashiro, D. J., et al. (1995). Identification of a patient with Bernard-Soulier syndrome and a deletion in the DiGeorge/velo-cardio-facial chromosomal region in 22q11.2. *Human Molecular Genetics, 4,* 763–766.

Croft, C. B., Shprintzen, R. J., Daniller, A. I., & Lewin, M. L. (1978). The occult submu-cous cleft palate and the musculus uvuli. *Cleft Palate Journal, 15,* 150–154.

de la Chapelle, A., Herva, R., Koivisto, M., & Aula, P. (1981). A deletion in chromosome 22 can cause DiGeorge syndrome. *Human Genetics 57,* 253–256.

DiGeorge, A. M. (1968). Congenital absence of the thymus and its immunologic con-sequences: Concurrence with congenital hypoparathyroidism. *Birth Defects Orig-inal Article Series, 4*(1), 116–121.

Down, J. L. H. (1866). Observations on an ethnic classification of idiots. *London Hospital Reports, 3,* 259–262.

Driscoll, D. A., Spinner, N. B., Budarf, M. L., McDonald-McGinn, D. M., Zackai. E. H., Goldberg, R. B., et al. (1992). Deletions and microdeletions of 22q11.2 in velo-cardio-facial syndrome. *American Journal of Medical Genetics, 44,* 261–268.

Edelmann, L., Pandita, R. K., Spiteri, E., Funke, B., Goldberg, R., Palanisamy, N., et al. (1999). A common molecular basis for rearrangement disorders on chromosome 22q11. *Human Molecular Genetics, 8,* 1157–1167.

Fisher, S. E., Vargha-Khadem, F., Watkins, K. E., Monaco, A. P., & Pembrey, M. E. (1998). Localisation of a gene implicated in a severe speech and language disorder. *Nature Genetics, 18,* 168–170.

Fokstuen, S., Vrticka, K., Riegel, M., Da Silva, V., Baumer, A., & Schinzel, A. (2001). Velo-facial hypoplasia (Sedláčková syndrome): A variant of velocardiofacial (Shprintzen) syndrome and part of the phenotypical spectrum of del 22q11.2. *European Jour-nal of Pediatrics, 160,* 54–57.

Fryburg, J. S., Lin, K. Y., & Golden, W. L. (1996). Chromosome 22q11.2 deletion in a boy with Opitz (G/BBB) syndrome. *American Journal of Medical Genetics, 62,* 274–275.

Giannotti, A., Digilio, M. C., Marino, B., Mingarelli, R., & Dallapiccola, B. (1994). Cayler cardiofacial syndrome and del 22q11: Part of the CATCH22 phenotype. *American Journal of Medical Genetics, 53,* 303–304.

Goldberg, R., Marion, R., Borderon, M., Wiznia, A., & Shprintzen, R. J. (1985). Pheno-typic overlap between velo-cardio-facial syndrome and the DiGeorge sequence. *American Journal of Human Genetics, 37,* A54.

Kaplan, E. N. (1975). The occult submucous cleft palate. *Cleft Palate Journal, 12*(4), 356–368.

Kinouchi, A., Mori, K., Ando, M., & Takao, A. (1976). Facial appearance of patients with conotruncal anomalies. *Pediatrics Japan, 17*(1), 84–87.

Lewin, M. L., Croft, C. B., & Shprintzen, R. J. (1980). Velopharyngeal insufficiency due to hypoplasia of the musculus uvulae and occult submucous cleft palate. *Plastic and Reconstructive Surgery, 65*, 585–591.

Lipson, A. H., Yuille, D., Angel, M., Thompson, P. G., Vanderwoord, J. G., & Beckenham, E. J. (1991). Velo-cardio-facial syndrome: An important syndrome for the dysmorphologist to recognize. *Journal of Medical Genetics, 28*, 596–604.

McDonald-McGinn, D. M., Emanuel, B. S., & Zackai, E. H. (1996). Autosomal dominant "Opitz" GBBB syndrome due to a 22q11.2 deletion. *American Journal of Medical Genetics, 64*, 525–526.

Meinecke, P., Beemer, F. A., Schinzel, A., & Kushnick, T. (1986). The velo-cardio-facial (Shprintzen) syndrome. Clinical variability in eight patients. *European Journal of Pediatrics, 145*, 539–544.

Merscher, S., Funke, B., Epstein, J. A., Heyer, J., Anne, P., Lu, M. M., et al. (2001). TBX1 is responsible for cardiovascular defects in velo-cardio-facial/DiGeorge syndrome. *Cell, 104*, 619–629.

Mitnick, R. J., Bello, J. A., Golding-Kushner, K. J., Argamaso, R. V., Shprintzen, R. J. (1996). The use of magnetic resonance angiography prior to pharyngeal flap surgery in patients with velo-cardio-facial syndrome. *Plastic and Reconstructive Surgery, 97*, 908–919.

Morrow, B., Goldberg, R., Carlson, C., Gupta, R. D., Sirotkin, H., Collins, J., et al. (1995). Molecular definition of the 22q11 deletions in velo-cardio-facial syndrome. *American Journal of Human Genetics, 56*, 1391–1403.

Robin, N. H., & Shprintzen, R. J. (2005). Defining the clinical spectrum of deletion 22q11.2. *Journal of Pediatrics, 147*, 90–96.

Scambler, P. J., Kelly, D., Lindsay, E., Williamson, R., Goldberg, R., Shprintzen, R. J., et al. (1992). Velo-cardio-facial syndrome associated with chromosome 22 deletions encompassing the DiGeorge locus. *Lancet, 339*, 1138–1139.

Sedláčková, E. (1955). Insufficiency of palatolaryngeal passage as a developmental disorder. *Časopis lékařů českých, 94*(12), 1304–1307.

Sedláčková, E. (1967). The syndrome of the congenitally shortened velum: The dual innervation of the soft palate. *Folia Phoniatrica, 19*(6), 441–450.

Séguin, E. (1846). *Le traitement moral, l'hygiene et l'education des idiots.* Paris: J. B. Bailliere.

Shprintzen, R. J. (1979). Hypernasal speech in the absence of overt or submucous cleft palate: The mystery solved. In R. Ellis & R. Flack (Eds.), *Diagnosis and treatment of palato glossal malfunction* (p. 37). London: College of Speech Therapists.

Shprintzen, R. J. (1997). Genetics, syndromes, and communication disorders. San Diego, CA: Singular.

Shprintzen, R. J. (2005). Velo-cardio-facial syndrome. In S. B. Cassidy & J. Allanson (Eds.), *Management of genetic syndromes* (2nd ed., pp. 615–632). New York: Wiley-Liss.

Shprintzen, R. J., Goldberg, R., Golding-Kushner, K. J., & Marion, R. (1992). Late-onset psychosis in the velo-cardio-facial syndrome. *American Journal of Medical Genetics, 42*, 141–142.

Shprintzen, R. J., Goldberg, R. B., Lewin, M. L., Sidoti, E. J., Berkman, M. D., Argamaso, R. V., et al. (1978). A new syndrome involving cleft palate, cardiac anomalies, typical facies, and learning disabilities: Velo-cardio-facial syndrome. *Cleft Palate Journal, 15,* 56–62.

Shprintzen, R. J., Goldberg R., Young. D., & Wolford, L. (1981). The velo-cardio-facial syndrome: a clinical and genetic analysis. *Pediatrics, 67,* 167–172.

Shprintzen, R. J., Schwartz, R., Daniller, A., & Hoch, L. (1985). The morphologic significance of bifid uvula. *Pediatrics, 75,* 553–561.

Shprintzen, R. J., Siegel-Sadewitz, V. L., Amato, J., & Goldberg, R. B. (1985). Anomalies associated with cleft lip, cleft palate, or both. *American Journal of Medical Genetics, 20,* 585–596.

Strong, W. B. (1968). Familial syndrome of right-sided aortic arch, mental deficiency, and facial dysmorphism. *Journal of Pediatrics, 73,* 882–888.

Tatum, S. A., III, Chang, J., Havkin, N., & Shprintzen, R. J. (2002). Pharyngeal flap and the internal carotid in velo-cardio-facial syndrome. *Archives of Facial and Plastic Surgery, 4,* 73–80.

Williams MA, Shprintzen RJ, Goldberg RB. (1985). Male-to-male transmission of the velo-cardio-facial syndrome: A case report and review of 60 cases. *Journal of Craniofacial Genetics and Developmental Biology, 5,* 175–180.

Wilson, D. I., Burn, J., Scambler, P., & Goodship, J. (1993). DiGeorge syndrome, part of CATCH 22. *Journal of Medical Genetics, 30,* 852–856.

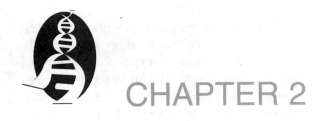

# CHAPTER 2

# The Expansive Phenotype of VCFS

*E*ssentially every organ, bodily function, and behavior can be affected in VCFS. The syndrome exhibits craniofacial, heart, brain, neurologic, limb, internal organ, genitourinary, skeletal, ocular, ear, vascular, glandular, dental, and muscle anomalies. These result in impairments of development, cognition and learning, mental health, speech and language, the immune system, the respiratory system, the endocrine system and growth, and the digestive system. It is possible that the reason that the large array of specific phenotypes has been reported in association with VCFS is that many people from many separate disciplines have studied the disorder. It is also possible that the deletion that causes the syndrome involves genes that are critical to embryonic development and postnatal function. Of course, these two factors are not mutually exclusive and both may be true. What is easy to understand is that by studying VCFS, clinicians and scientists may be able to unlock some of the mysteries of how specific genomic elements result in some common human illness, both physical and mental.

The first step in the process is to understand the full expanse of the phenotype in VCFS. This next section of the text will detail the phenotype of VCFS by categories of anomalies that occur in VCFS with a frequency higher than would be expected in the general population. To date, 190 distinct anomalies or patterns of anomalies have been described.

Because VCFS has so many clinical findings, referrals to care providers tend to be based on presenting symptoms. A pediatric cardiologist and cardiothoracic surgeon are often the first contact for babies with the syndrome. Developmental delay may prompt referral to a variety of early intervention specialists including speech pathologists, physical therapists, and occupational therapists. Developmental pediatricians may be also be in the picture, and if seizures present, a child neurologist. Immune disorders will result in an immunology evaluation and hypocalcemia an endocrine workup. Hypernasality and articulation impairment will bring the patient to a speech pathologist and perhaps a cleft palate team and an otolaryngologist and reconstructive surgeon. If the syndrome is not known to them, each of these specialists will manage these disorders in the manner they might for others who do not have VCFS. They would also not refer the patient for additional investigations to rule out other problems associated with VCFS, such as renal anomalies, tethered spinal cord, and vascular anomalies. Each specialist would take care of his or her corner of the syndrome and may not appreciate the bigger picture. The purpose of this chapter is to describe in great detail the phenotypes associated with VCFS and how they may interrelate with other anomalies associated with the syndrome. The categories and specific anomalies associated with VCFS will be used as a template for quick referral. We will number each anomaly consecutively and the entire list will be available in the Appendix.

## CRANIOFACIAL ANOMALIES

The following craniofacial malformations and variants have been reported in association with VCFS:

1. Palate anomalies, including overt cleft palate, submucous cleft palate, occult submucous cleft palate, deficient muscle, and asymmetric palate

2. Asymmetric pharynx

3. Platybasia

4. Retrognathia

5. Asymmetric crying facies (infancy)

6. Functional facial asymmetry

7. Structural facial asymmetry

8. Straight facial profile

9. Hypotonic facies

10. Vertical maxillary excess

11. Small primary teeth

12. Enamel hypoplasia (primary dentition)

13. Downturned oral commissures

14. Microstomia

15. Microcephaly

16. Small posterior cranial fossa

17. Cleft lip

## Palatal Anomalies

It has been reported that approximately 75% of individuals with VCFS have structural anomalies of the palate (Shprintzen, 1999; Shprintzen, 2005a) and essentially the same percentage has velopharyngeal insufficiency (Shprintzen, 1999). The anomalies of the palate in VCFS can be divided into the following types.

### *Overt Cleft Palate*

Overt clefts of the palate are the least common type of palate anomaly in VCFS. In a sample of 815 individuals with VCFS ascertained from our own clinical cases and from members of The Velo-Cardio-Facial Syndrome Educational Foundation, Inc. in response to a questionnaire study, we found that only 18% had overt palatal clefts (Figure 2–1), and of those, the majority were clefts of the soft palate only. Moreover, a large number of the overt clefts were part of the Robin sequence because of the association of cleft palate with retrognathia and upper airway obstruction (Williams, Shprintzen, & Goldberg, 1985).

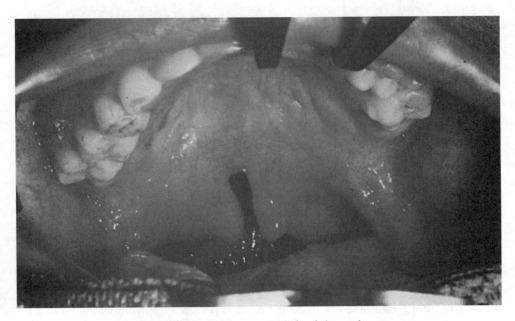

**FIGURE 2–1.** An overt cleft of the velum.

## Submucous Cleft Palate

Nearly half of individuals with VCFS have submucous clefts of the palate (Golding-Kushner, 1991; Shprintzen, 1999) that could be detected orally by the presence of a bifid uvula with or without other stigmata such as a notch in the posterior border of the hard palate and zona pellucida (Figure 2–2). Very few individuals with VCFS have the classic triad of submucous cleft palate (bifid uvula, zona pellucida, and notched hard palate). Most have bifid uvulas or even notched or boxy uvulas (Figure 2–2) without other palatal stigmata detectable on oral examination.

## Occult Submucous Cleft Palate

As described earlier in Chapter 1, occult submucous cleft palate was originally described in individuals obviously affected with VCFS although the syndrome had not yet been delineated (Kaplan, 1975). Occult submucous cleft palate cannot be detected without an endoscopic view of the nasal surface of the velum and this can be problematic in children with VCFS who are often

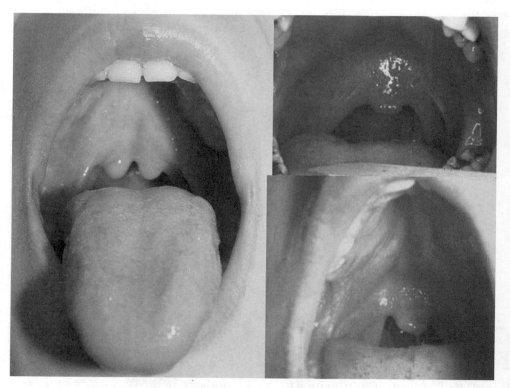

**FIGURE 2–2.** Examples of submucous cleft palate in individuals with VCFS.

fearful of nasopharyngoscopy. Because of the behavioral patterns of VCFS that can include generalized anxiety, impulsivity, and phobias, many clinicians may choose to defer, delay, or even forego nasopharyngoscopy because of the difficulty involved or their fear that they may traumatize the child. However, the importance of endoscopic examination cannot be emphasized enough. Besides showing the midline depression of the palate representing absence of the musculus uvulae, the examination can also show severely ectopic internal carotid arteries and laryngeal anomalies (Video 2–1).

The anomalies of the velum in occult submucous cleft can be subtle, ranging from a prominent midline depression to a gentle concavity to a flat nasal surface of the velum (Figure 2–3). When seen in a lateral view videofluoroscopy, the velum is short and thin (Golding-Kushner, 1991; Shprintzen, 1982), and during speech, it does not thicken, as would a normal palate (Figure 2–4). In the normal palate, the thickening of the velum during speech is caused by the presence of the musculus uvulae (Figure 2–5). The contraction of the musculus uvulae causes it to thicken at its belly because it has no firm attachment at its distal end where it ends in the blind sac of the uvula. In VCFS, the musculus uvulae is absent so that there is no thickening of the velum with palatal motion. The shortness of the velum plus increased volume in the pharynx (to be discussed later) makes the palate appear very short and thin (Golding-Kushner et al., 1991) within the confines of a large pharynx (Video 2–2). It is also possible that the thinness of the palate often observed in VCFS (Golding-Kushner, 1991; Shprintzen, 1982) is related to generalized thinning of the pharyngeal muscles (Golding-Kushner, 1991) caused by abnormalities of the muscle fibers at the cellular level Zim et al., 2003), rather than to a cleft, per se.

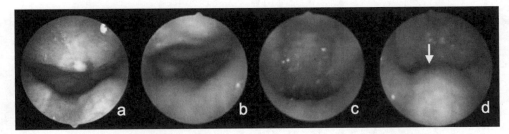

**FIGURE 2–3.** Endoscopic view of the nasal surface of the velum in three patients with VCFS compared to a normal individual (*right*). At the *far left* (**a**) is a child with VCFS and occult submucous cleft palate showing a deep midline groove in the velum. At *middle left* (**b**), the nasal surface of the velum in a child with VCFS and occult submucous cleft showing a gentle midline concavity, and at *middle right* (**c**) is a child with VCFS and occult submucous cleft palate with a flat velum. The normal (**d**) shows a prominent convexity in the midline of the velum (*arrow*) representing the musculus uvulae.

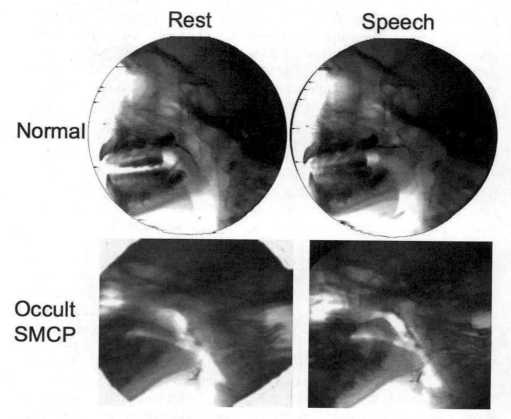

**FIGURE 2–4.** Lateral view videofluoroscopy in a 5-year-old with a normal palate (*top row*) and a 5-year-old with VCFS who has an occult submucous cleft palate (*bottom row*) at rest and during phonation of /pa-pa-pa/. Note that the normal palate thickens considerably during phonation, whereas the palate with an occult submucous cleft elevates but does not thicken at all.

## Asymmetric Palate

A more recently reported structural and functional anomaly of the palate (and pharynx) is asymmetry (Chegar, Tatum, Marrinan, & Shprintzen, 2006). In an endoscopic and fluoroscopic study of 121 subjects with VCFS, 67% were found to have asymmetric elevation (Video 2–3) of the velum during speech and the position, length, and size of the levator veli palatini was found to be asymmetric in many cases. The velar midline was also found shifted to one side or the other (Figure 2–6).

One study suggested that structural palatal anomalies occur in only 14% of cases, 9% cleft palate and 5% submucous cleft palate (Ryan et al., 1997), a clear error probably based on ascertainment parameters and a failure to recognize more subtle anomalies of velar structure. Data for the Ryan et al. study

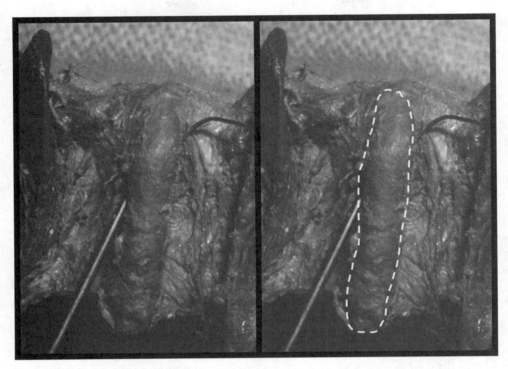

**FIGURE 2–5.** A normal musculus uvulae in a cadaver dissection.

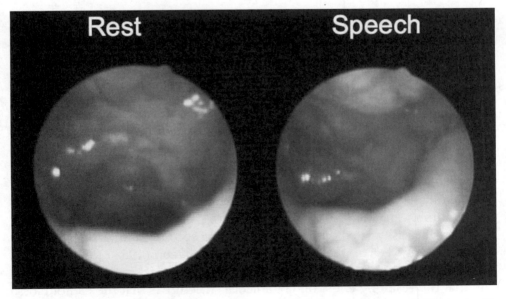

**FIGURE 2–6.** Asymmetric palate at rest and during speech in an individual with VCFS and occult submucous cleft palate.

were obtained from more than 20 centers in Europe. There was no reported attempt to confirm examiner reliability or validity. Occult submucous cleft palate was not a recognized clinical finding in any cases, although it was noted that 32% had velopharyngeal insufficiency. The structural findings were not discussed. A major percentage of the sample was children ranging in age from 0 to 5 years. It is not known how many of these subjects were infants and were therefore not speaking so that velopharyngeal insufficiency could not be determined. Asymmetry of the palate was also not mentioned as a clinical finding in this study, which preceded the report of Chegar et al. (2006).

## Asymmetric Pharynx

Chegar et al. (2006) also reported that the pharynx was commonly asymmetric in VCFS. Asymmetric structure of the posterior pharyngeal wall or movement of the lateral pharyngeal walls was seen in 76% of people with VCFS (Video 2–4). Endoscopic observation showed that one side of the pharynx had more fullness than the other with the right side showing that increased fullness more frequently than the left. The increased unilateral fullness often compromised the pyriform sinus tract on that side, potentially resulting in restriction of the flow of liquids and food to the cricopharyngeus, resulting in coughing or choking. Asymmetric lateral pharyngeal wall motion (Video 2–5) is also common among cases in which there is any degree of active medial movement (most individuals with VCFS have little or no lateral wall movement).

## Platybasia

Platybasia refers to an abnormally obtuse angle of the skull base. The human cranium has a flexion along the skull base that differentiates the anterior portion of the cranium that supports the facial bones and the posterior aspect that contains the posterior portions of the brain and the junction with the spinal cord (Figure 2–7). The angulation of the skull base is typically analyzed by measuring the angle from the nasion (the junction of the nasal bones to the frontal bone of the calvarium) to the sella turcica (the bony projection containing the pituitary gland) to the basion (the anteriormost point of the foramen magnum). This angle is typically about 128° with a standard deviation of approximately 4°. The implications of platybasia cut across several of the anomalies associated with VCFS by creating secondary anomalies that may not be primary gene effects. Arvystas and Shprintzen (1984) found that the skull base angulation in VCFS was significantly more obtuse than in normals and that the resulting effect on craniofacial structure is that the glenoid fossa and the temporomandibular joint are more posteriorly located than in the normal (Figure 2–7), so that the mandible is retropositioned (retrognathia). Retrognathia can lead to Robin sequence, malocclusion, and possible airway

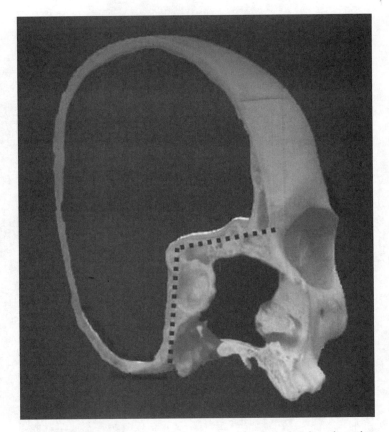

**FIGURE 2–7.** Drawing of the human cranium showing the flexion point in the skull base.

obstruction in infancy. Arvystas and Shprintzen (1984) also found that the obtuse angulation of the skull base caused the posterior skull base to move backwards with resulting deepening of the pharynx, because the posterior pharyngeal wall is attached to the prevertebral fascia and suspended from the posterior skull base. The increase in pharyngeal depth is an additional factor in the frequency and severity of velopharyngeal insufficiency in VCFS (Figure 2–8). The posterior rotation of the skull base also causes a secondary anterior displacement of the forehead because of the counterclockwise rotation of the cranium around the flexion point at the base (Figure 2–9). With the forehead displaced anteriorly, the upper eyelids become stretched in the same direction making them look "puffy" or hooded in relation to the globe. Although the malar bones and maxillary basal bone are actually normal in VCFS, the cheeks look flat because the forehead is in a more anterior position in relation to the malar eminences. Therefore, the reported flattening of the midface in VCFS is actually an optical illusion of relative projection of structures in the profile view (Figure 2–9). At this point, it is not known if the flattening of the skull base is a primary feature of skeletal formation in VCFS or secondary

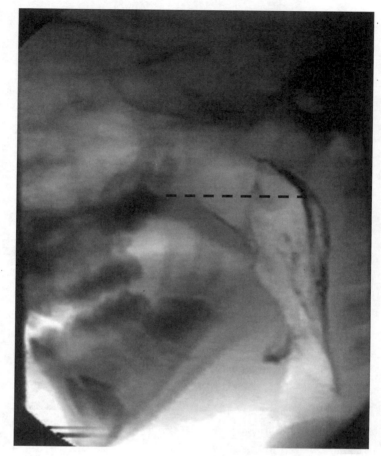

**FIGURE 2–8.** Increased pharyngeal depth in VCFS related to platybasia.

to reduced volume of the cerebellum. It is possible that cerebellar hypoplasia results in decreased pressure on the embryonic and postnatal skull base so that there is reduced mechanical force driving it forward (Figure 2–10). Skull growth is driven in part by bone growth potential, but also by the internal forces of a growing brain that are pushing the cranium from within, therefore driving growth of the bones and remodeling of their architecture based on the needed size for the brain within the cranial fossa.

## Retrognathia

Abnormal position of the mandible and retrusion of the chin can be caused by three different factors: micrognathia, retrognathia, and microretrognathia. Micrognathia refers to a small or hypoplastic mandible. Micrognathia can be caused by a small body of the mandible, by a short ascending ramus, or both.

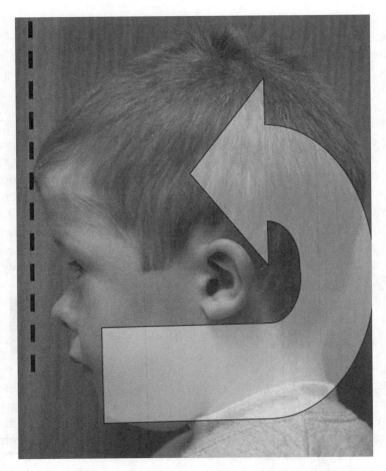

**FIGURE 2–9.** Counterclockwise rotation of the cranium in VCFS resulting in anterior displacement of the forehead.

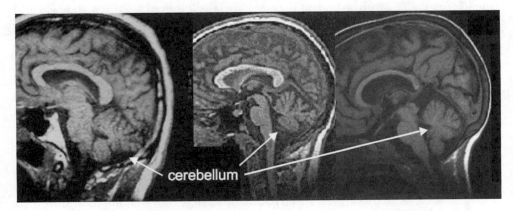

**FIGURE 2–10.** Cerebellar hypoplasia may reduce pressure on the skull base, therefore decreasing anterior movement of the posterior basicranium.

Individuals with VCFS do not typically have micrognathia. They have retrognathia, an abnormal retruded position of the mandible. The size and architecture of the mandible are normal in VCFS (Arvystas & Shprintzen, 1984), although the chin looks retrusive. In VCFS, the abnormal position of the mandible is related to retrognathia secondary to platybasia as discussed above. Microretrognathia is the combination of a small mandible and retrognathia. Although micrognathia is not a syndromic feature of VCFS, one must keep in mind that children with VCFS also inherit all of the other genes from their parents. Their physical appearance is not completely related to the deletion. It is therefore possible for micrognathia to be inherited as a separate trait from one or both parents who may have it. It is important to distinguish between micrognathia and retrognathia because of the prognosis for future growth of the lower jaw. Micrognathia implies that the mandible has fewer cells to begin with and with time the amount and pattern of growth will remain the same or get worse. It will certainly not be normal. In retrognathia with a structurally normal mandible, normal growth should be anticipated.

## Asymmetric Crying Facies

The majority of diagnoses of VCFS are being made because there is routine screening of children born with severe conotruncal heart anomalies such as interrupted aortic arch type B, tetralogy of Fallot, and truncus arteriosus. Although individuals with VCFS constitute a large percentage of each of these major heart anomalies (50% of interrupted aortic arches, 25% of tetralogies, and over 50% of truncus cases), the majority of children with VCFS do not have these serious heart anomalies. The most common heart malformation in VCFS is ventricular septal defect, and many children with VCFS will have other more minor heart anomalies, such as atrial septal defect, aortic valve anomalies, or other aortic arch anomalies. It is also true that approximately 25–30% of children with VCFS have no congenital heart disease. Therefore, a question that is often asked is if there are any clinical features that should present as diagnostic "red flags" for VCFS in the neonatal period. One such red flag is asymmetric crying facies (Figure 2–11). Asymmetric crying facies typically refers to an abnormal lack of movement of one side of the mouth, usually the lower lip and corner of the mouth on the same side, during crying when it is most obvious. The combination of asymmetric crying facies with congenital heart disease has been referred to by some as Cayler syndrome (Cayler, 1969). It has since been learned that the association of asymmetric crying facies and congenital heart disease is most often associated with VCFS and that patients previously diagnosed with Cayler syndrome have the same 22q11.2 deletion (Bawle, Conard, Van Dyke, Czarnecki, & Driscoll, 1998). If a newborn is noted to have asymmetric crying facies in addition to chronic nasal regurgitation, VCFS becomes a highly probable diagnosis and these findings would be sufficient to warrant a FISH study.

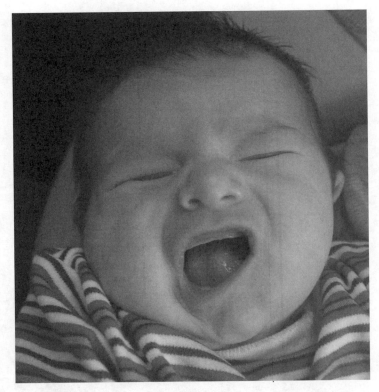

**FIGURE 2–11.** An infant with VCFS and asymmetric crying facies.

## Functional Facial Asymmetry

Although asymmetric crying facies can be easy to detect in neonates, facial asymmetry may manifest itself in a more subtle manner in VCFS. Asymmetric crying facies involves an obvious lack of movement in the lower part of the face on one side. Some individuals with VCFS do not have an obvious asymmetric face during crying, but do have asymmetry of smile or normal facial animation during speech and emotional expression (Figure 2–12). Because facial expression is something that evolves over time, such minor asymmetries may not become obvious until early childhood.

## Structural Facial Symmetry

A small percentage of individuals with VCFS have asymmetry of the face that is based on skeletal growth (Figure 2–13). Although structural facial asymmetry is not a common feature of VCFS, it does occur in approximately one fifth of affected individuals (Shprintzen, 1999). Facial asymmetry is a common cranio-facial malformation and is found in oculo-auriculo-vertebral spectrum (also

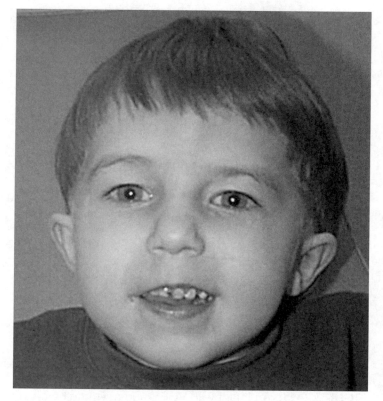

**FIGURE 2–12.** Subtle asymmetry of facial animation during smiling in VCFS.

known as hemifacial microsomia), branchio-oto-renal syndrome (BOR syndrome), X-linked mental retardation, and Dubowitz syndrome, just to name a few. All of these syndromes have some clinical overlap with VCFS such as cervical spine anomalies, hearing loss, renal anomalies, developmental delay, cognitive impairment, and relatively small stature in childhood. It is therefore not uncommon for VCFS to be misdiagnosed in the absence of major heart anomalies that are most easily recognized as being associated with VCFS.

## Straight Facial Profile

As mentioned earlier, the anomaly of the skull base in VCFS results in alterations of position of the facial bones including the mandible and maxilla. These alterations do not represent malformations of the facial bones, but rather an appearance caused by relative positions of the facial bones to one another. The midface and resulting facial profile appear flat because they are more recessed than normal in relation to the forehead. With the forehead more in

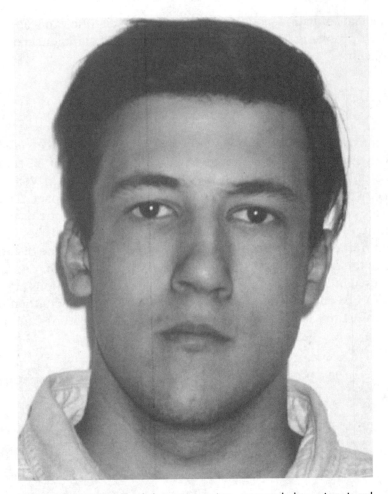

**FIGURE 2–13.** Facial asymmetry caused by structural abnormality. Note that the chin point is skewed to the right and that the right side of the face is concave while the left is convex.

advance of the facial bones than normal, the midface looks deficient in relation to the prominent upper third of the skull. However, the facial bones themselves are normal.

### Hypotonic Facies

Facial muscle tone is reduced in VCFS, as is generalized muscle tone in the extremities. Decreased facial muscle tone is variable in VCFS and does not result in a complete lack of facial movement or expression, but there is reduced facial animation, and the decrease in muscle tone can lead to secondary growth problems. This facial hypotonia is not of sufficient magnitude to affect speech.

### Vertical Maxillary Excess

Vertical maxillary excess, sometimes referred to as *long face syndrome*, is most likely not a primary malformation in the syndrome, but is secondary to the hypotonia that is a common, nearly constant finding in VCFS. Vertical maxillary excess is a longer than normal lower third of the face. The mature human face can be divided into thirds, the upper face being the distance from the hairline to the nasal root, the middle third being the distance from the nasal root to the base of the nose, and the lower third being the distance from the base of the nose to the chin point. In the normal face, the thirds are approximately equal in length (Figure 2–14). At birth, facial proportions are typically normal in VCFS and it is time and growth that yield vertical lengthening of the lower third of the face. Hypotonia of the facial musculature can cause this

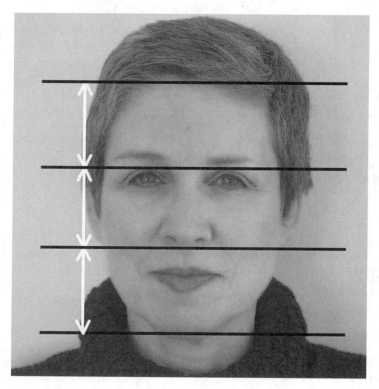

**FIGURE 2–14.** The normal mature human face with the thirds demarcated, showing that the thirds are of approximately equal length.

type of lengthening based on the functional matrix model of facial growth postulated by Moss (Moss, 1975; Moss & Rankow, 1968). The functional matrix model predicates craniofacial growth on a balance of internal and external forces on the bones of the cranium and face that cause the bones to remodel and follow particular growth paths based on those forces. These forces include oral and nasal airflow, the muscular forces of the tongue internally, and the muscles of the lips, cheeks, and neck externally. If there is any type of imbalance or abnormality in any of these forces, facial growth will be redirected in an abnormal vector. There is ample experimental evidence to support the functional matrix model, including the results of animal studies (Vargervik, Miller, Chierici, Harvold, & Tomer, 1984) and human studies (Woodside, Linder-Aronson, Lundstrom, & McWilliam, 1991) that have shown that alteration of respiratory pattern from normal nasal breathing to persistent mouth breathing causes transverse maxillary collapse, anterior skeletal open-bite, and vertical lengthening of the face. In VCFS, hypotonia reduces the internal force applied by the muscles of the facial envelope (lips and cheeks). This often results in a mouth-open posture, especially during sleep. With the mouth open, the mandible grows in a more vertical direction (Figure 2–15). With the mouth open more than normal, there is also an increase in the growth of the alveolar bone of the maxilla resulting in what many people refer to as "a high arched palate." The increase in alveolar bone growth is caused by the mouth-open posture (Figure 2–16). As the dentition erupts into the maxillary arch and the roots of the maxillary teeth lengthen, it is necessary for them to be firmly embedded in alveolar bone. The teeth in the upper dental arch continue to erupt until they come into contact with the teeth of the lower arch. Once they do contact the mandibular teeth, signals generated by the dental nerves cause the eruption of the teeth to stop. If the mouth is in a persistently open position, the maxillary teeth cannot contact their mandibular

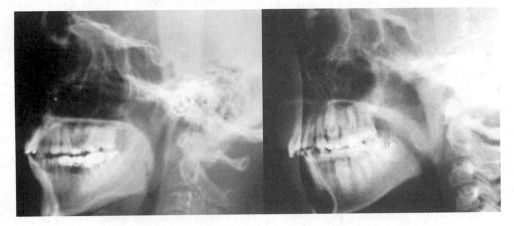

**FIGURE 2–15.** Cephalometric radiographs comparing normal growth (*left*) to a vertical pattern (*right*).

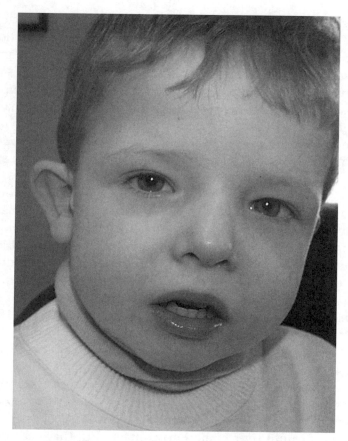

**FIGURE 2–16.** Mouth-open posture in VCFS.

counterparts and therefore keep erupting. In order for the roots of the maxillary teeth to remain embedded in bone, more alveolar bone is deposited around them causing vertical lengthening of the maxilla. The lengthening of the maxilla, being in the alveolar bone, is below the level of the nasal base, thus increasing the length of the lower third of the face.

## Small Primary Teeth and Enamel Hypoplasia

Although dentition is generally grossly normal in VCFS, there are some minor variations that are present in both the primary and secondary dentition, although the problems are more significant in the primary teeth. The primary teeth in children with VCFS tend to be slightly smaller than in other children, although this difference is not severe. Hypomineralization and enamel hypoplasia are also present, and this probably results in the smaller tooth size (Klingberg, Oskarsdottir, Johannesson, & Noren, 2002; Klingberg et al., 2005).

## Downturned Oral Commissures

Downturning of the corners of the mouth is common in VCFS and is partly related to hypotonia, and partly to mandibular position. With the mandible more retropositioned, the corners of the mouth are stretched downward, and with the decrease in overall muscle tone, the effect on the facial musculature will be more pronounced.

## Microstomia

Microstomia (Figure 2–17) is a relatively common finding in VCFS. In infancy, the association of microstomia with characteristic ears and congenital heart disease, cleft palate, or Robin sequence should strongly raise the suspicion of VCFS as the primary diagnosis. If the corners of the mouth do not extend considerably past the base of the nose on each side, then the mouth is small (microstomia), and while this is a minor anomaly that does not require treatment, it is often of diagnostic significance.

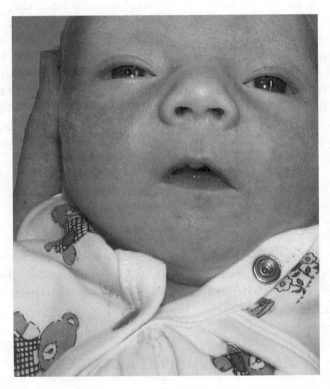

**FIGURE 2–17.** Microstomia in VCFS. Note that the corners of the mouth at rest do not extend beyond the alar cartilages of the nose laterally.

## Microcephaly

Microcephaly, a small head circumference, is found in approximately a quarter of patients with VCFS (Shprintzen, 1999). Microcephaly has been correlated with reduced brain size, developmental delay, and mental retardation, but this relationship, although a positive correlation, is not perfect (Camp, Broman, Nichols, & Leff, 1998). Studies from several laboratories have shown a reduction of brain volume in VCFS that is correlated on a population basis with reduced IQ scores, but head circumference was not analyzed in these reports (Eliez, Schmitt, White, Wellis, & Reiss, 2001; Kates et al., 2004). Microcephaly can be caused by reduced brain volume (primary microcephaly) or by craniosynostosis (premature fusion of the skull bones) related to bone formation abnormalities (secondary microcephaly). Craniosynostosis is not a clinical feature of VCFS.

## Small Posterior Cranial Fossa

The posterior cranial fossa is the portion of the cranium that contains the cerebellum, medulla, and other brain structures. It is the portion of the cranium posterior to the flexion of the skull base behind the sella turcica. Hypoplasia of the cerebellum has been reported in VCFS (Eliez et al., 2001; Mitnick, Bello, & Shprintzen, 1994). Specifically, the cerebellar vermis has been found to be smaller than normal in VCFS and this may be related to abnormal social cognition (Eliez et al., 2001) and poor coordination (Mitnick et al., 1994). It is not clear at the present time if the small size of the posterior cranial fossa is related to the small size of the cerebellum's resulting failure to push the calvarial bones outward and the posterior cranial base downward causing platybasia. This type of response to a small cerebellar volume would be consistent with the functional matrix model.

## Cleft Lip

The first case of cleft lip associated with VCFS was published by Lipson et al. (1991). Since that report, several more cases have been documented. Although cleft lip is an uncommon finding in VCFS, it does occur with higher frequency than in the general population and it is therefore a low frequency anomaly in the syndrome.

# EAR AND HEARING ANOMALIES

The external ears in VCFS have a characteristic appearance that is not typically abnormal. However, the structure of the auricles is characteristic of the syndrome because of a number of normal variants that can be excellent diagnostic clues. In some cases, there are a number of anomalies of the external ears and the auditory system that are clearly abnormal, but such cases are in the minority. The auditory system has been implicated as a target of the effects of hemizygosity of *TBX1* based on animal studies that resulted in both external and inner ear anomalies (Arnold et al., 2006), but there is not strong evidence that the same malformations occur in humans. Anomalies noted in affected humans include:

18. Overfolded helix

19. Attached lobules

20. Protuberant, cup-shaped ears

21. Small ears

22. Mildly asymmetric ears

23. Frequent otitis media

24. Mild conductive hearing loss

25. Sensorineural hearing loss

26. Ear tags or pits

27. Narrow external ear canals

## Overfolded Helix

The helical rims are overfolded and are often adherent to the ear in a high percentage of individuals with VCFS. Nearly 60% of individuals with VCFS have markedly overfolded helices (Shprintzen, 1999) and more than 85% have some overfolding (Figure 2–18). There are two possible explanations for this

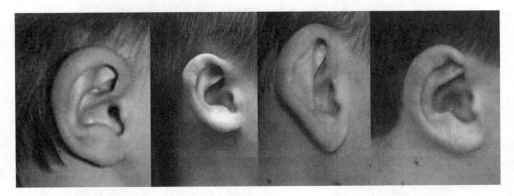

**FIGURE 2–18.** Overfolding of the helices and characteristic ear morphology in VCFS ranging from mild to severe.

overfolding. One is that one or more of the deleted genes affects ear formation as suggested by Arnold et al. (2006). Another is that the helices are overfolded because of poor peripheral perfusion. As will be discussed later, individuals with VCFS have smaller blood vessels, especially in the periphery, and many have congenital heart disease that reduces peripheral perfusion. As the ears form in the embryonic period, they unfurl almost like a rubber raft being filled with air. This unfurling is driven by perfusion, with the blood pumping through the small vessels in the ear to drive its growth outward. The weaker the perfusion, the less the unfurling, resulting in overfolding of the helices.

### Attached Lobules

Attached ear lobes are not abnormal. They are found in at least 10% of the general population. However, the lobules are attached to the side of the head in the large majority of people with VCFS, probably over 80% (Figure 2–19). Although not an abnormal trait, the presence of this variation of normal seems to have some significance in the process of embryonic development, and because it is such a consistent finding it is likely to be related to the deletion.

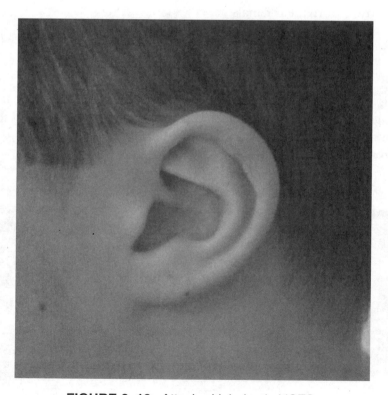

**FIGURE 2–19.** Attached lobules in VCFS.

## Protuberant, Cup-Shaped Ears

Protuberant ears (Figure 2–20) have been reported to occur in approximately half of individuals with VCFS (Shprintzen, 1999). Protuberant ears are also common in the general population, although not at the rate of 50%. However, protruding ears are common among individuals with low muscle tone, because the muscles that are attached to the auricles in the lateral aspects of the head are weaker than normal. Protuberant ears in VCFS are likely to be secondary to hypotonia.

## Small Ears

The ears in people with VCFS are often small and more than two standard deviations below the mean for length based on population norms (Figure 2–21). Even when ears are within normal limits for size, they tend to be smaller than the average length for age. It is possible that the reduced length of the ear is

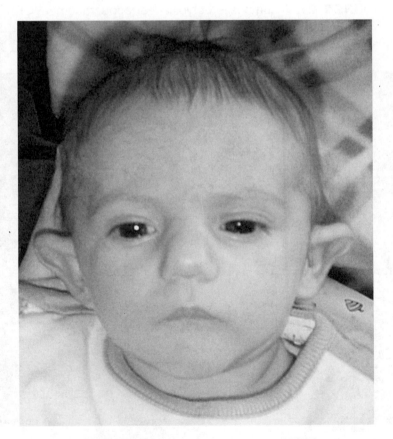

**FIGURE 2–20.** Protuberant ears in VCFS.

related to the characteristics of the ear mentioned above, specifically the overfolding of the helices and attached lobules. If the helical rims are not unfurled and the lobules are not dangling below the point of attachment to the head, then the ears will lose at least 5 mm of vertical length. In some cases, the ears are extremely small and somewhat malformed, but such cases are unusual (Figure 2-22).

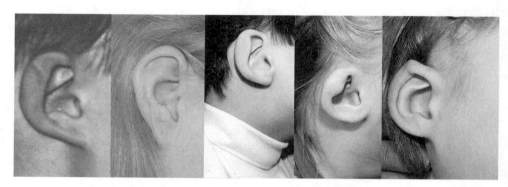

**FIGURE 2–21.** A composite of typical ear appearance in VCFS.

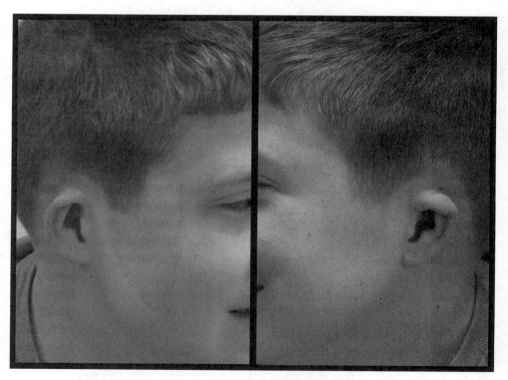

**FIGURE 2–22.** Very small and mildly malformed ears in VCFS.

Clinical descriptions of VCFS often cite "low set ears." Low set ears are not a feature of VCFS. In fact, because of platybasia, the position of the ears in VCFS is typically normal if not a bit higher than normal. In some rare cases of VCFS where there is severe webbing of the neck (to be discussed later), the ears may be in a lower position than is typical, but such cases are unusual. The reason some clinicians may misinterpret ear position in VCFS is because of the size of the ears and the overfolding of the helices. When the helices are significantly overfolded, the upper poles of the auricles are shorter than normal. This shortness of the upper portion of the ear may make it appear to be low set, but this is merely an optical illusion. The position of the external auditory canal is the true determining factor in terms of ear position, and this is not low in VCFS.

## Mildly Asymmetric Ears

Facial asymmetry has already been described, and in such cases, the ears are typically asymmetric, although the correlation between structural facial asymmetry and ear asymmetry is not perfect. Structural asymmetry of the ears is seen in approximately 15% of individuals with VCFS (Shprintzen, 1999). The discrepancy is often in size only, but there may also be a difference in form (Figure 2–23).

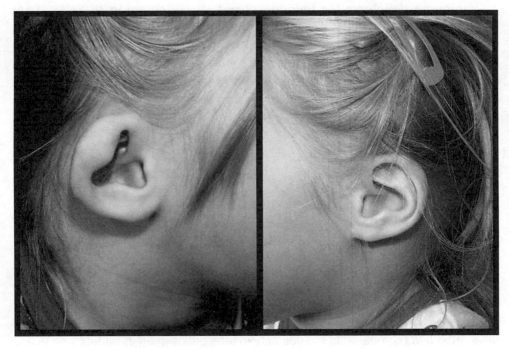

**FIGURE 2–23.** Asymmetric ears in VCFS.

## Frequent Otitis Media

Chronic serous otitis media and acute otitis media with middle ear effusion is common in children with VCFS, although not universal (Gereau et al., 1988b). Unlike children with isolated clefts of the palate, the reasons for chronic middle ear disease in VCFS are multifactorial and include abnormalities of the nasopharyngeal eustachian tube orifice, abnormal placement of the muscles that dilate the eustachian orifice, and immune disorders or immune deficiency. The eustachian orifice in VCFS is malformed in much the same way as in individuals with cleft palate (Shprintzen & Croft, 1981). The torus tubarius is more compressed and the orifice smaller than normal (Figure 2–24). In addition, the dilator of the nasopharyngeal end of the eustachian tube is the levator veli palatini muscle (Video 2-6). The belly of the levator veli palatini is normally positioned underneath the torus tubarius, the cartilage that surrounds the eustachian orifice in the nasopharynx. During swallowing and speech, the contraction of the levator impulses the torus upward, causing the orifice to dilate (Video 2-6). It has been demonstrated that the eustachian tube cartilage is abnormal in individuals with cleft palate (Dickson, 1976; Shprintzen & Croft, 1981). The torus tubarius is compressed and the orifice is smaller than normal (Dickson, 1976). The belly of the levator is displaced anteriorly so that when the levator contracts, the belly of the muscle fills and occludes the orifice rather than dilating it (Video 2-7). The same anomalies of the eustachian tube are present in VCFS resulting in both a structural and functional obstruction of the eustachian tube.

Immune deficiency or immune disorders are common in VCFS. True immune deficiency is not a frequent finding in VCFS, but when it does occur,

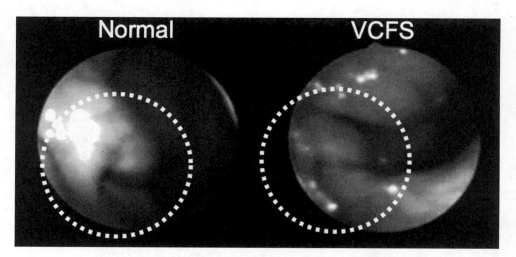

**FIGURE 2–24.** Endoscopic view of the nasopharyngeal orifice of a normal eustachian tube (*left*) compared to the eustachian tube orifice in an individual with VCFS and occult submucous cleft palate (*right*).

chronic middle ear disease is a nearly universal outcome, as is chronic upper and lower respiratory disease. More common is an immune disorder that may or may not be accompanied by positive laboratory findings such as reduced T-cell populations. In cases of immune disorder, children with VCFS get more frequent upper respiratory infections than other children and more frequent middle ear disease. In such cases, it is recommended that antipneumococcus vaccines such as Prevnar and Pneumovax be administered in childhood. In addition to the protection against pneumonia that these vaccines provide, they also reduce the frequency of middle ear disease.

Some clinicians and researchers believe that reflux may account for middle ear disease in some cases by contaminating the eustachian tube so that bacteria can travel in a retrograde fashion from the pharynx to the middle ear. The landmark study by Bluestone (1971) considered the issue of eustachian tube function in children with cleft palate. The study demonstrated the absence of retrograde contamination of the middle ear in children with clefts. Based on the malformations of the eustachian tube cartilage documented by Dickson (1976) and Shprintzen and Croft (1981) with the orifice of the eustachian tube so significantly compromised, it is unlikely that reflux contributes to middle ear disease in individuals with VCFS. This link has not been confirmed scientifically. Clinical experience has demonstrated that the frequency of chronic middle ear disease in VCFS occurs as frequently in patients who do not have GERD as in those who do.

## Mild Conductive Hearing Loss

Conductive hearing loss in VCFS is typically transient, fluctuating, and mild as is often found in individuals with cleft palate. The frequency of this type of hearing loss is similar to that found in cases of nonsyndromic cleft palate (Gereau et al., 1988b). Structural anomalies of the middle ear are not common in VCFS. However, attention to middle ear disease in VCFS is important, and taking a "wait and see" approach is potentially dangerous because risk of immune disorder may predispose the patient to a worsening and progressive condition, including the potential for cholesteatoma.

## Sensorineural Hearing Loss

Although sensorineural hearing loss is not a common finding in VCFS, it does occur with a slight increase in frequency above that seen in the general population. Approximately 10% of individuals with VCFS have sensorineural hearing loss, and in most cases, the hearing loss is mild to moderate and unilateral. Several cases of severe or profound hearing loss have been reported (Reyes, LeBlanc, & Bassila, 1999), but it is possible that some of these patients may have other etiologies for their hearing loss, such as a connexin 26 mutation

(Venail et al., 2004), that would be expected to occur with the same frequency among individuals with VCFS as in the general population.

It is interesting to note that a high percentage of those cases with sensorineural hearing loss are unilateral, and the majority of those are left-sided by a two-to-one margin. In most genetic hearing losses of sensorineural origin, the hearing loss is typically bilateral and relatively symmetric. It has been suggested that many anomalies in VCFS are secondary to vascular disruptions (Shprintzen, Morrow, & Kucherlapati, 1997), and this type of unilateral sensorineural hearing loss may be indicative of that type of problem.

### Ear Tags or Pits

Although not a common finding in VCFS, ear tags and ear pits have been found in a number of cases that exceeds the frequency of this minor anomaly in the general population. The implication of ear pits in the general population, however, is different than it is in VCFS. When ear tags or pits are found in individuals who do not have VCFS, clinicians would typically check for other signs consistent with oculo-auriculo-vertebral dysplasia (also known as hemifacial microsomia), such as conductive hearing loss, ocular dermoids, facial asymmetry and mandibular structure, and cervical spine anomalies. With the exception of ocular dermoids (also known as choristomas), the other anomalies associated with oculo-auriculo-vertebral dysplasia also commonly occur in VCFS. In other words, there is phenotypic overlap between VCFS and oculo-auriculo-vertebral dysplasia, although they are two separate and distinct disorders.

### Narrow External Ear Canals

A high percentage of children with VCFS have very narrow ear canals. It is likely that this reduction in diameter of the ear canals occurs secondary to the skull base anomalies in the syndrome. The obtuse angle of the basicranium rotates the base of the skull upward, therefore reducing the overall height of the ear canal and possibly the middle ear space as well. Reduced volume of the ear canal can create problems in otoscopic examination and hearing testing with either tympanometry or otoacoustic emissions.

## THE NOSE

All of the characteristic nasal findings in VCFS are actually variants of normal and not anomalies. Although the nose has a characteristic appearance, it is a variable feature that can be affected by age, sex, ethnic background, and epigenetic factors. The nasal characteristics include:

28. Prominent nasal bridge

29. Vertically long nose

30. Bulbous nasal tip

31. Mildly separated nasal domes (tip appears bifid)

32. Pinched alar base, narrow nostrils

33. Narrow nasal passages

### Prominent Nasal Bridge (Nasal Root)

The nasal root (the bridge of the nose) appears more prominent in VCFS than in most people (Figure 2-25), although prominent nasal bridges are not uncommon in the general population. This characteristic appearance is not at all anomalous and has little or nothing to do with the embryologic formation of the nose. The prominence of the nasal root, the point where the nasal

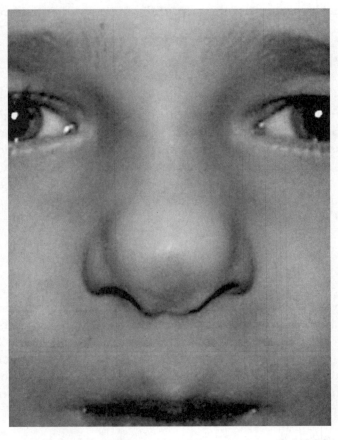

**FIGURE 2–25.** Prominence of the nasal root in VCFS.

bones join the forehead at the glabella, is related to the same rotational growth pattern of the skull caused by platybasia. As was discussed earlier, the counterclockwise posterior rotation of the basicranium causes the forehead to be more anteriorly positioned. If the forehead is more anterior than normal the nasal root that joins the forehead at the glabella must also come forward, making it look more prominent.

### Vertically Long Nose

The length of the nose is increased in VCFS, as is the entire middle portion of the face. Vertical maxillary excess is typically accompanied by increased length of the nose because the nasal bones are an integral part of the entire maxilla. Functionally, this increased length is of no significance.

### Bulbous Nasal Tip

The nasal tip in VCFS is large compared to most people and is prominent and round or bulbous. The rounded nasal tip appears prominent because it is accentuated by the narrowness of the base of the nose and the pinched nasal alae.

### Mildly Separated Nasal Domes (Tip Appears Bifid)

Because the nasal tip is large and broad, the domes of the alar cartilages are further apart than normal, resulting in a depression in the center of the nose (Figure 2–26). Some people mistakenly believe that this separation of the nasal domes represents a malformation or bifurcation of the nose. It does not, and this type of nasal tip is common among people who have broad nasal tips. The well-known French actor, Gérard Depardieu (Figure 2–26, right), has this type of nasal tip, and if one pays attention to people they pass on the street, he will see this type of nasal tip with some frequency.

### Pinched Alar Base, Narrow Nostrils

There is narrowing of the entire middle of the face in VCFS. Some of this appearance is secondary to the vertical maxillary excess that is often related to collapse of the maxillary arches. The maxilla constitutes the floor of the nose, so any constriction of the maxillary arch will have the effect of narrowing the nasal base and nostrils (Figure 2–27). In cases with microstomia, narrowing of the alar base is to be expected in relation to the size of the entire nasomaxillary complex.

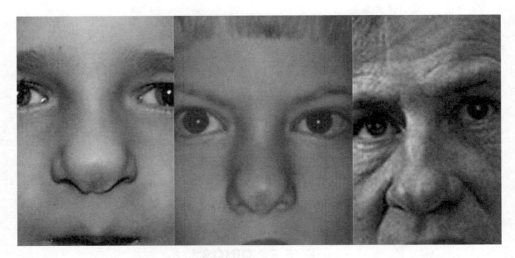

**FIGURE 2–26.** Separation of the domes of the nasal alae resulting in the appearance of a bifurcation of the nasal tip (*left and center*). Notice, however, that this type of appearance of the nasal tip does occur in the general population in individuals with similar nasal anatomy (*right*), indicating that this is simply a variant of normal.

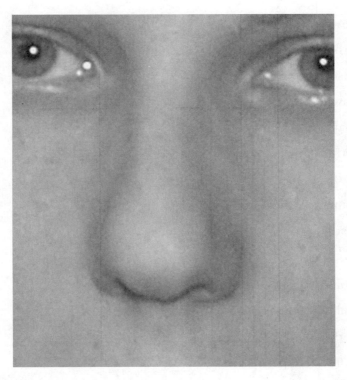

**FIGURE 2–27.** Pinched alar base and narrow nostrils in VCFS.

## Narrow Nasal Passages

Similar to narrowing of the floor of the nose, the entire nasal passage will be narrowed if the maxillary arch is constricted. The floor of the nose will constrict if the maxilla has any degree of collapse and this will have the effect of bringing the nasal turbinates together, therefore narrowing the nasal airway. In addition, chronic nasal congestion secondary to chronic upper airway disease will cause chronic enlargement of the turbinates and constriction of the nasal airway.

## EYE FINDINGS

Anomalies of the eye are often considered to be important in understanding the developmental mechanisms of syndromes. The eyes form from outpouchings of the developing prosencephalon of the embryonic brain. Therefore, links between eye anomalies and underlying brain malformations are often suspected. The significance of these correlations in VCFS is not yet known, nor are the genetic contributions to them. Included among eye findings in VCFS are:

34. Tortuous retinal vessels

35. Suborbital congestion ("allergic shiners")

36. Strabismus

37. Narrow palpebral fissures

38. Puffy upper eyelids

39. Posterior embryotoxon

40. Small optic disk

41. Prominent corneal nerves

42. Cataracts

43. Iris nodules

44. Iris coloboma (uncommon)

45. Retinal coloboma (uncommon)

46. Small eyes

47. Mild orbital hypertelorism

48. Mild vertical orbital dystopia

### Tortuous Retinal Vessels

Anomalies of the retinal vessels have long been considered to be related to congenital heart disease, although the causal relationship was never known and was only hypothesized to be related to abnormalities in perfusion. Ophthalmologists have classically been trained to recognize the association between tortuous retinal vessels and congenital heart disease. However, in VCFS, it has been found that even in cases where there is no congenital heart disease present, the retinal vessels are tortuous (Mansour, Wang, Goldberg, & Shprintzen, 1987). It is therefore likely that the ocular vascular anomalies in VCFS (Figure 2–28) are not secondary to congenital heart disease but are part of a more general problem with angiogenesis.

### Suborbital Congestion ("Allergic Shiners")

Dark circles under the eyes can be related to skin pigmentation, but in VCFS, the darkening seen in the suborbital region is related to peripheral venous congestion of the small vessels under the eyes (Figure 2–29). In the general

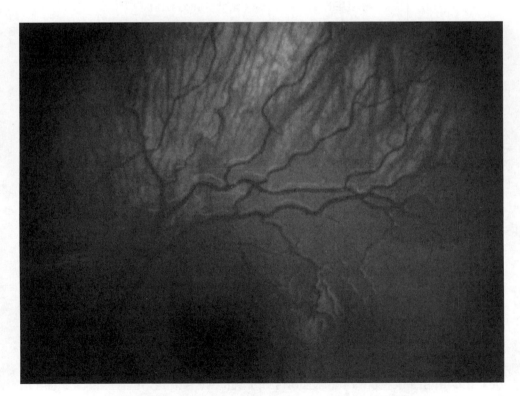

**FIGURE 2–28.** Retinal vessel anomalies in VCFS.

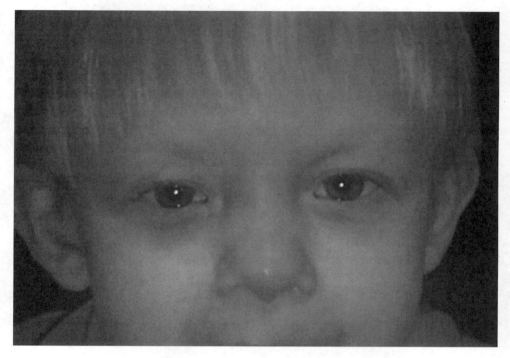

**FIGURE 2–29.** Suborbital congestion.

population, this type of suborbital congestion is common in people with upper respiratory allergies and can be caused by irritation of the eyes with constant tearing and subsequent rubbing of the eyes. The suborbital soft tissues become inflamed and congested. In VCFS, this appearance has no relation to allergies or illness. The frequency of suborbital congestion is the same in people with VCFS who have chronic upper airway irritation and those who do not. It is likely that the anomaly is caused by a narrow caliber of the blood vessels (to be discussed later) and abnormalities of the platelets (also to be discussed later), which can cause congestion of the very tiny surface vessels under the eyes where the skin is thin and subcutaneous features are easily visible. Although noticeable, this feature does not cause any problems or create any risks.

## Strabismus

Strabismus (Figure 2–30) may present as an esotropia (when one eye turns in) or exotropia (when one eye turns out). Strabismus is common among children who have hypotonia. It is also common if there is abnormal vision in one eye or if the brain's perception of vision from that eye is abnormal. This can lead to amblyopia, where the brain essentially shuts off the vision in one eye in order

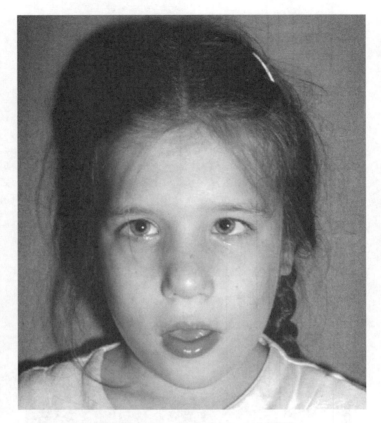

**FIGURE 2–30.** Strabismus in VCFS.

to prevent competing visual signals from each eye. Strabismus can sometimes be corrected early by using spectacles to refocus one eye, but surgery is often necessary to correct an eye muscle imbalance.

### Narrow Palpebral Fissures

In the initial description of VCFS (Shprintzen et al., 1978), vertical shortening of the palpebral fissures was mentioned as a clinical finding. Some have mistakenly thought that this reference was to horizontal shortening of the palpebral fissures, meaning that the eyes appeared small in overall circumference. The actual appearance is that the eyes appear more like they are squinting. Other labels for the same appearance of the eyes are *puffy eyelids* or *hooded eyelids* (Figure 2–31). The soft tissue above the eyes appears redundant because, as was mentioned in the section on skull anatomy, the forehead is positioned slightly more forward than normal. The anterior positioning of the forehead draws the superior orbital rims forward so that the eyelids are suspended in

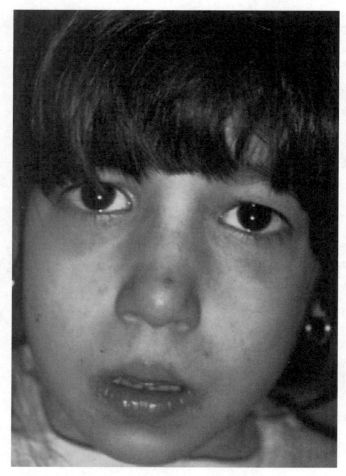

**FIGURE 2–31.** Puffy or hooded upper eyelids.

a more anterior position than normal, resulting in the next clinical feature on the list, puffy (or hooded) upper eyelids. The effect in terms of appearance is to make the eyes look smaller than normal in the vertical dimension.

## Puffy (Hooded) Upper Eyelids

Following the same of reasoning as detailed above, the eyelids look puffier or hooded because they extend more forward of the globe of the eye than normal because of the anterior positioning of the supraorbital ridges. The upper lids therefore drape forward rather than straight over the eye. This is not an actual anomaly of the eyelids, but rather a secondary soft tissue arrangement in relation to skull morphology.

## Posterior Embryotoxon

Posterior embryotoxon is considered to be a developmental anomaly of the anterior chamber of the eye. It presents as an opacification of the margin of the cornea. Posterior embryotoxon is known to be associated with a number of multiple anomaly syndromes including VCFS and Allagile syndrome. However, it is also found in 6 to 15% of otherwise normal people. Posterior embryotoxon does not cause any visual impairment, although it is thought to be a predictor of eventual glaucoma. However, there is no known increase in glaucoma in people with VCFS.

## Small Optic Disk

In a paper published by Fitch (1983), the first report of eye anomalies in VCFS reported a case with small optic disks. In reports that followed, small optic disk was found to belong to a broader range of eye anomalies that included optic nerve anomalies and small eyes. These findings are of significance because embryologically, the eyes are actually an outpouching of the developing diencephalon, and some eye anomalies are considered predictors of underlying brain malformations. When the optic disk is small, the implication is that the optic nerve is small. The optic disk is the part of the optic nerve that joins the back of the retina where the retinal ganglion cell axons enter the optic nerve. The optic nerve, although referred to as a cranial nerve, is more accurately a portion of the central nervous system similar to the spinal cord. Therefore, anomalies of the optic nerve are often consistent with structural malformations of the brain. Although there has not yet been specific research to correlate optic nerve anomalies to brain anomalies in VCFS, it is understood that developmental brain anomalies are common in the syndrome.

## Prominent Corneal Nerves

Mansour et al. (1987) reported prominent corneal nerves in VCFS. The corneal nerves that make the cornea sensitive to touch are not typically visible on routine ophthalmoscopic examination, but are visible when the nerves are labeled as prominent. Prominent corneal nerves have been associated with a number of genetic syndromes including neurofibromatosis type 1, Noonan syndrome type 1, Bannayan-Riley-Ruvalcaba syndrome, and myotonic dystrophy type 1. Prominent corneal nerves are often considered to be indicative of keratoconus, an ophthalmic disease that can be progressive and result in visual impairment. Although we have seen this diagnosis made in VCFS, we are unaware of any significant visual impairments in the syndrome.

## Cataracts

Cataracts are a common finding in the general population, but typically with advancing age. Congenital or early onset cataracts have been seen in a small number of patients with VCFS. This is a low frequency anomaly in the syndrome, and because it is uncommon, the causes for it in VCFS are unknown.

## Iris Nodules

Iris nodules are incidental findings in a number of genetic disorders and have typically been associated with neurofibromatosis type 1 (NF1). Nodules in the iris probably represent some type of developmental anomaly of the eye but, to date, there is no evidence for the specific cause in VCFS. Although found in VCFS, they do not impair vision.

## Iris and Retinal Coloboma

Iris and retinal colobomas will be considered together because they often occur together as part of the same fusion anomaly of the eye. The eye and its components form by a tubular fusion process that occurs in a circular direction much like the formation of the neural tube. The final fusion point is at the bottom of the eye in the 6 o'clock position. The iris is most commonly affected and is easily visible to clinical examination (Figure 2–32). In order to

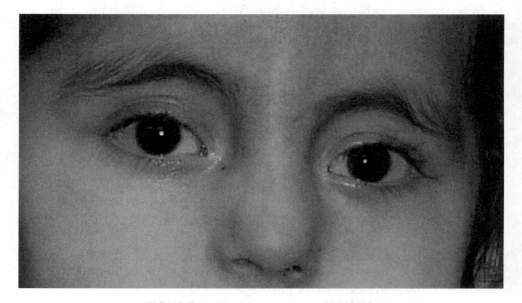

**FIGURE 2–32.** Iris coloboma in VCFS.

detect a retinal coloboma, a full ophthalmologic assessment is required. Iris colobomas are strongly indicative of underlying optic nerve and brain anomalies, and therefore iris colobomas raise additional suspicions. Retinal colobomas are of interest in VCFS in part because of their strong association with another syndrome associated with rearrangements of chromosome 22 known as cat-eye syndrome (CES). CES is caused by a partial trisomy or partial tetrasomy of chromosome 22 that includes part of the short arm and the same 22q11.2 region that is deleted in VCFS. Other clinical features of CES include many of the same findings characteristic of VCFS, including conotruncal heart anomalies, cleft palate, developmental delay, retruded lower jaw, and renal anomalies. Although there is no similarity in facial appearance, clinicians unfamiliar with the phenotypes of the syndromes might confuse the two. Fortunately, the diagnostic procedure FISH would detect either syndrome, with VCFS showing deletion from one copy of chromosome 22 at the q11.2 band and CES showing extra copies of the region.

## Small Eyes

In some cases of VCFS, probably less than 10%, the eyes are actually small by measurement. As with small optic disks and iris/retinal colobomas, small eyes can be indicative of underlying anomalies of the brain. Hypoplasia of the eyes can reflect hypoplasia of the underlying forebrain. To date, investigators have not correlated eye size with cognitive function or brain volume.

## Mild Orbital Hypertelorism

Orbital hypertelorism is an increased distance between the eyes. When the eyes are actually wide spaced because of increased distance between the orbits, the measurements from the inner corners of the eye (the inner canthus) and the outer corner of the eyes (outer canthus) are both increased. If only the inner canthus measurement is greater than normal, the condition is known as telecanthus. In telecanthus, the eyes are normally placed on the skull, but there may be increased tissue along or near the inner corner, such as epicanthal folds or a thickened nasal bridge. In VCFS, those patients who have wide-spaced eyes tend to have mild orbital hypertelorism (Figure 2–33), although some cases have mild telecanthus related to the increased width of the nasal root. Hypertelorism is not a common finding in VCFS, but it does occur in approximately 12% of the clinical case load at the International VCFS Center in Syracuse. This is a far higher percentage than seen in the general population. The occurrence of orbital hypertelorism in VCFS has led to some considerable confusion in the diagnosis of the syndrome and phenotypic overlap with other syndromes, as discussed in Chapter 1 in relation to Opitz syndrome, sometimes referred to as the Opitz G/BBB syndrome.

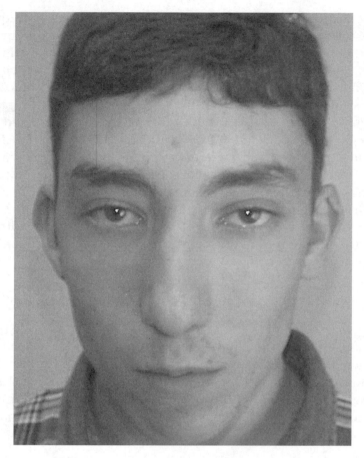

**FIGURE 2–33.** Orbital hypertelorism in VCFS.

## Mild Vertical Orbital Dystopia

Orbital dystopia refers to asymmetric placement of the orbits on the face. The position of the orbits can be altered by a number of abnormalities, some congenital malformations, and some secondary positional deformations. Some individuals with VCFS have vertical orbital dystopia (Figure 2–34). In some cases, the dystopia is related to the structural asymmetry of the face discussed previously in this chapter. In other cases, it may be related to positional plagiocephaly, a common problem in hypotonic infants. Babies with VCFS have low muscle tone, and many spend a major portion of their early weeks or months after birth lying on their backs because of prolonged illnesses or hospitalizations for surgery. Babies often develop a "most comfortable position" and will tend to lie in that posture for most of their sleep. With the infant skull soft and the brain growing actively, the constant external pressure on one spot from lying in that position will redirect growth in the opposite direction. The

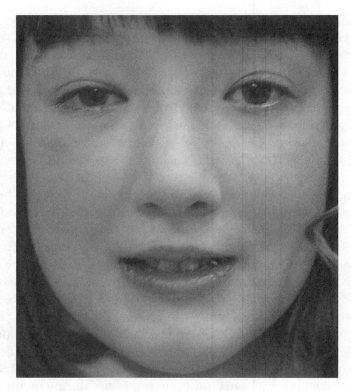

**FIGURE 2–34.** Orbital dystopia in VCFS.

cranium becomes asymmetric and the orbits located at the base of the cranium will respond by being positioned in relation to the asymmetric cranium. In some rare cases, dystopia can be related to severe hypoplasia of one side of the brain, resulting in abnormal internal growth forces on the cranium, which results in asymmetry.

## CARDIAC FINDINGS

Heart anomalies and malformations of the major blood vessels leading to and from the heart are found in approximately 71% of individuals with VCFS (Shprintzen, 1999). The most common heart malformation found in VCFS is ventricular septal defect (VSD), although in many instances the VSD is found in association with other heart anomalies. However, VSD without other major heart anomalies is still a common finding in VCFS and is also among the most common anomalies in humans in general.

Although VSD is the most common heart anomaly in VCFS, it is not known what percentage of VSDs are found in people with VCFS. For less common major complex cardiac anomalies such as tetralogy of Fallot, truncus arteriosus, and interrupted aortic arch type B, people with VCFS constitute the largest etiology of these malformations. VCFS is the largest single cause of complex anomalies derived from the embryonic conotruncus, the portion of the developing heart that becomes the outflow portions of the ventricles, and the truncus arteriosus that becomes the ascending aorta and pulmonary trunk. Approximately half of all individuals born with interrupted aortic arch type B and slightly less than half born with truncus arteriosus have VCFS (Goldmuntz et al., 1998). At least 15% of people born with tetralogy of Fallot have VCFS (Goldmuntz et al., 1998), and this percentage increases when right-sided aortic arch is present.

Although most of the congenital heart problems in VCFS can be surgically repaired, many without long-term risks, some of the anomalies do increase the risk of developing a condition known as subacute bacterial endocarditis (SBE). SBE is an infection of the heart's valves that can develop as a result of bacteria entering the bloodstream from an injury elsewhere in the body, such as the gingiva (gums), nasal passages, or urinary tract. Depending on the type of congenital heart anomaly present, it may be necessary to take antibiotics prior to certain medical or dental procedures to protect against SBE (known as SBE prophylaxis). The conditions warranting SBE prophylaxis and the type of antibiotic coverage required are occasionally revised by medical authorities, so it is important to check with an individual's cardiologist before procedures where bleeding might occur because of injury during medical or dental examination or therapy. Therefore, prior to endoscopies or dental treatment (as examples), cardiologists should be consulted about the need for SBE prophylaxis. Although SBE is not specific to VCFS and not a feature of the syndrome per se, children with VCFS can be prone to this problem, especially if their immune function is abnormal.

The full range of heart anomalies associated with VCFS includes:

49. VSD (ventricular septal defect)

50. ASD (atrial septal defect)

51. Pulmonic atresia or stenosis

52. Tetralogy of Fallot

53. Right-sided aorta

54. Vascular ring

55. Patent ductus arteriosus (PDA)

56. Interrupted aortic arch, type B

57. Coarctation of the aorta

58. Double aortic arch

59. Aortic valve anomalies

60. Aberrant subclavian arteries

61. Truncus arteriosus

62. Anomalous origin of carotid artery

63. Transposition of the great vessels

64. Tricuspid atresia

### Ventricular Septal Defect (VSD)

VSD is the most common type of congenital heart malformation and is one of the most common anomalies in humans. VSD is a hole in the septum that separates the two lower chambers of the heart (Figure 2–35) known as the ventricles. There are three different types of VSDs, depending on their position. A VSD that occurs in the membranous portion of the ventricular septum is known as a perimembranous VSD, and these are the most common type and they do occur in VCFS. A second type occurs in the muscular portion of the septum. A third type known as a conoseptal defect is related to abnormality of the outlet tract. VSDs can be related to a malalignment of the septal components, and such malalignment defects are common in VCFS. VSDs can close spontaneously after birth when they are initially small. When present, VSDs

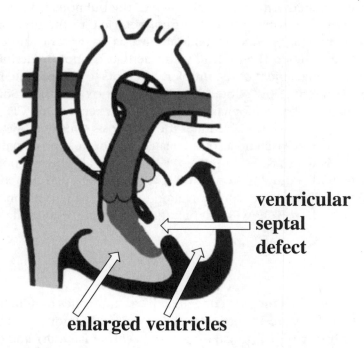

**ventricular septal defect**

**enlarged ventricles**

**FIGURE 2–35.** Ventricular septal defect.

can increase the risk of bacterial endocarditis, necessitating the use of prophylactic antibiotics for dental work or endoscopies. When the VSD is large,
blood from the left ventricle, which is oxygen rich, mixes with blood from
the right ventricle, which is oxygen depleted. That blood then recirculates
through the lungs even though it already has picked up oxygen from the
lungs before it was returned to the left ventricle from the pulmonary veins.
Because some oxygen-rich blood displaces oxygen-depleted blood, the heart
has to work harder to oxygenate all of the blood, and if it fails to do so
because of the VSD, the blood remains oxygen depleted causing cyanosis.

### Atrial Septal Defect (ASD)

ASD is a less common anomaly in children with VCFS than VSD, but it does
occur as the only intracardiac heart anomaly in some children and in combination with other heart anomalies in others. An ASD is an opening in the septum
that divides the two upper chambers of the heart. When large enough, blood
shunts from one upper chamber to the other so that a portion of the oxygen-
depleted blood bypasses the lungs. When the amount of shunt is small, ASDs
may be asymptomatic, but large ASDs cause blood to be depleted of oxygen.

### Pulmonic Stenosis or Atresia

Narrowing, malformation, or absence of the pulmonary valve prevents blood
from flowing normally from the right ventricle to the pulmonary artery and
then to the lungs. When pulmonic atresia is present, there is a complete
blockage of blood flow to the ventricle that cannot be definitively repaired.
Surgical management of the problem attempts to compensate for the blockage
by rerouting the flow of blood to allow better oxygenation. Surgical outcomes
for congenital heart anomalies in general are excellent in VCFS, but pulmonary
atresia or severe stenosis reduces the prognosis considerably (Anaclerio et al.,
2004). Pulmonary stenosis or atresia is present in approximately one third of
individuals with VCFS (Shprintzen, 1999). It has also been reported that among
people with complex congenital heart disease such as tetralogy of Fallot
(TOF), VCFS is more common among those with pulmonary atresia than
those who have TOF without pulmonary atresia (Goldmuntz et al., 1998).

### Tetralogy of Fallot (TOF)

TOF is a form of complex congenital heart anomalies that includes the following clinical features: ventricular septal defect, pulmonary stenosis, right ventricular hypertrophy (thickening of the ventricular wall), and overriding aorta
(the aorta is positioned over the VSD so that the aortic valve is open to both

the right and left ventricle instead of the right ventricle alone (Figure 2–36). The exact position of the aorta determines the amount of mixing of blood from the right and left ventricles, and this can be quite variable, thus affecting the severity of the clinical symptoms. Also important to the degree of effect on the newborn's health is the severity of the VSD, the severity of the pulmonic stenosis, and the degree of right ventricular hypertrophy. The presence of pulmonary atresia significantly worsens the prognosis and the effect on the child's health. TOF is common in VCFS, but more importantly, of children born with TOF, approximately 15% have VCFS. Therefore, children born with TOF are routinely given FISH tests for a 22q11.2 deletion unless they have another recognizable syndrome that has TOF as a common finding, such as Down syndrome.

### Right-Sided Aorta

The aortic arch normally rises and descends to the lower portion of the body on the left side of the heart. In VCFS, the aortic arch often descends on the right side, crossing over to the left well below the heart, or begins on the right side and crosses over to the left near or at the level of the heart. When the

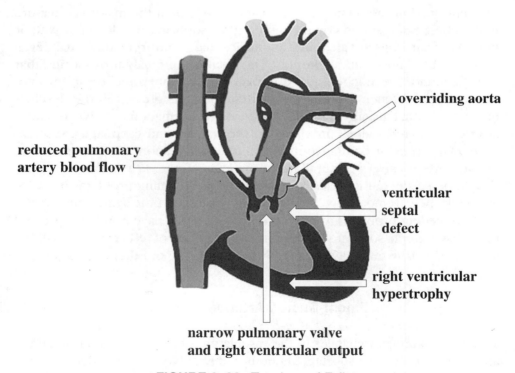

**FIGURE 2–36.** Tetralogy of Fallot.

aorta crosses over to the left in proximity to the esophagus and trachea, it can cause compression of one or both of these tubes, thereby having an impact on breathing and eating. If other major thoracic vessels, such as the right subclavian artery, are also anomalous, a vascular ring may form around the trachea causing severe respiratory compromise. Vascular rings are relatively common in VCFS. Feeding may be affected because compression of the esophagus prevents the entire bolus of swallowed food, including liquids, from reaching the stomach. If a portion of the bolus is hung up in the esophagus, it is typically regurgitated in order to clear the esophagus and relieve it of abnormal pressure. This reflexive response is often misconstrued as reflux or even acalasia, when in reality it is simply a normal response to a structural esophageal constriction. Although the constriction caused by the anomalous aorta may resolve with age and expansion of the chest as growth occurs, in some cases the condition is permanent and causes persistent problems into adult life. In cases where the right-sided aorta does not impinge on the esophagus or trachea, it is asymptomatic and will not be detected without imaging studies. Right-sided aortic arch may occur in VCFS in the absence of other heart anomalies, but it may also occur in association with other heart anomalies including VSD and TOF (Young, Shprintzen, & Goldberg, 1980).

## Vascular Ring

As mentioned in the section above, rearrangements of the major vasculature in the chest can result in compression of the esophagus, the lower airway, or both. Vascular rings are anatomic anomalies that result from abnormal development of the aortic arch complex. The resulting anomaly forms a ring that can surround the trachea and esophagus. The embryonic error involves abnormal persistence of some vascular components present in the developing embryo that usually disappear later, or malformations of two or more arteries that are in close proximity to the trachea and esophagus. Vascular rings may occur in combination with intracardiac anomalies, but may also occur without any structural malformations of the heart. Vascular rings should be suspected in cases of swallowing or breathing problems in VCFS, although they are not very common malformations in the syndrome. Breathing and feeding problems in VCFS do not necessarily have a single cause and rarely have simple solutions. For example, a diagnosis of reflux (GER or GERD) is not necessarily mutually exclusive of vascular ring or other anomalies.

## Patent Ductus Arteriosus (PDA)

There are significant changes in the vasculature of a fetus and that of a child after birth. There are a substantial number of fetal blood vessels that are present prior to birth but that disappear in late fetal life or shortly after birth. One example is the ductus arteriosus, a fetal blood vessel that connects the aorta to the pulmonary artery. A patent ductus arteriosus (PDA) is the persistence of this embryonic circulation, which has the effect of mixing the oxygen-rich blood from the aorta with the oxygen-depleted blood of the pulmonary artery. The shunting of blood from the aorta to the pulmonary artery also has the effect of increasing blood pressure in the pulmonary artery (pulmonary hypertension), a potentially dangerous complication. The ductus arteriosus is a necessary component of fetal circulation and has no negative effect on oxygenation because the lungs do not serve that purpose until birth, when the lungs fill with air for the first time.

## Interrupted Aortic Arch, Type B

More than half of all babies born with interrupted aortic arch, type B (IAA, type B), have VCFS (Goldmuntz et al., 1998). Today, surgical correction of IAA is possible, but at the time VCFS was first described, few if any babies survived attempts to surgically repair this problem. This anomaly is exactly what its name implies. There is a lack of development of the aorta resulting in a complete lack of circulation through the aorta to the rest of the body below the point of interruption. Type B IAAs are located proximal to the left subclavian artery. If a PDA is present (see above), then there is an outlet for some oxygenated blood to reach the lower body until it closes. The high frequency of VCFS among individuals with IAA, type B clearly mandates screening of all babies born with IAA, type B unless they have another recognizable syndrome that causes this anomaly, such as Down syndrome.

## Coarctation of the Aorta

Coarctation refers to a narrowing of the aorta, usually just past the region where the major chest arteries branch off from it. This narrowing is variable in degree and only in the mildest of cases is treatment unnecessary. Aortic arch anomalies are found in the majority of individuals with VCFS. Coarctation of the aorta is not the most common of these anomalies in VCFS, but its presence in a newborn, especially when present in association with other anomalies such as asymmetric crying facies or nasal emesis, should prompt the recommendation for a FISH study.

## Double Aortic Arch

This anomaly of the aortic arch involves a splitting of the main aortic branch into two ascending arteries that can then form a vascular ring around the esophagus and/or trachea, resulting in breathing difficulties, swallowing problems, or both. This anomaly may not present a hemodynamic problem and therefore may go undetected if the resultant feeding and breathing problems are not surmised to be related to a possible vascular ring. This presents a particularly difficult problem of differential diagnosis in VCFS where feeding and breathing problems have many possible etiologies.

## Aortic Valve Anomalies

The aortic valve regulates blood flow from the left ventricle to the aorta. The normal aortic valve consists of three leaflets embedded in a ring of fibrous tissue, allowing the outflow of blood from the heart, but not inflow. A bicuspid aortic valve has only two leaflets, and these are often thicker than the normal valve and less flexible so that the outflow of blood meets more resistance than normal. Bicuspid aortic valve is one of the most common congenital heart anomalies in humans, estimated to occur in as many as 1:50 newborns, but it is not one of the more common heart anomalies in VCFS. Other aortic valve anomalies in VCFS include aortic valve stenosis and regurgitation (McElhinney et al., 2003).

## Aberrant Subclavian Arteries

The subclavian arteries, as the name implies, are major blood vessels that arise from the aorta and run horizontally under each clavicle to the arms. Aberrant subclavian arteries are common in VCFS and may occur without structural heart anomalies. An aberrant right subclavian can be seen when the aorta is left-sided and an aberrant left subclavian is seen when the aortic arch is right-sided. In both of these types of aberrant arteries, the subclavian can course behind the esophagus, causing compression of the esophagus. Symptomatically, "spitting up" or emesis is seen in such cases and is often mislabeled as reflux. Actually, the bolus of food or liquid never reaches the stomach and, after sitting in the constricted esophagus for a short while, the natural response is for a reverse peristalsis of the esophagus to clear it, resulting in emesis. In cases of reflux or persistent emesis, vascular compressions of the esophagus should be suspected.

## Truncus Arteriosus

Truncus arteriosus is an uncommon complex congenital heart anomaly, but it is important to note that a very high percentage of patients with truncus arteriosus have VCFS (Goldmuntz et al., 1998), perhaps more than half. Individuals with truncus arteriosus have one large single great vessel at the top of the heart (a truncus) instead of two (the aorta and the pulmonary artery). There is typically a large ventricular septal defect underneath the truncus. The truncus carries blood to the body and the lungs at the same time rather than one vessel going to the lungs (the pulmonary artery) and one to the body (the aorta). Unless early surgery is done to separate the flow of blood to the body from the flow to the lungs, high blood pressure can damage the pulmonary arteries.

### Anomalous Origin of Carotid Artery

The carotid artery is the source of many anomalies in VCFS, including the common carotid and the internal carotid arteries. The origin of the paired common carotid from the aorta may be abnormal in VCFS, and many variants of an anomalous origin of the carotid exist. Carotid anomalies are often incidental findings associated with structural anomalies of the heart.

### Transposition of the Great Vessels

The *great vessels*, sometimes called the *great arteries*, refers to the aorta and the pulmonary artery. The normal arrangement of the great vessels is that the pulmonary artery arises from the right ventricle where it takes the oxygen-depleted blood to the lungs, and the aorta arises from the left ventricle where it takes the oxygen-rich blood to the body. In transposition of the great vessels, the aorta and pulmonary artery are attached to the wrong ventricles, so that the aorta arises from the right ventricle taking oxygen-depleted blood to the body, while the pulmonary artery arises from the left ventricle taking already oxygenated blood to the lungs. This switch of blood flow is life threatening. If there is a mechanism for mixing of oxygenated blood with oxygen-depleted blood, such as a large VSD or ASD, then the situation may not be as severe, and if a PDA is present, this will also allow for some oxygenated blood to reach the body. However, in all cases, surgical switching of the arteries becomes necessary at some point.

### Tricuspid Atresia

The tricuspid valve controls the flow of blood from the right atrium to the right ventricle, where it is then circulated to the lungs via the pulmonary artery. Tricuspid atresia is the absence of the tricuspid valve, and this prevents blood flow from the right atrium to the right ventricle, leaving the right ventricle hypoplastic. The presence of an atrial septal defect and a ventricular septal defect allows blood to return to the right atrium through the atrial septal defect and into the left atrium, where it can mix with oxygen-rich blood from the lungs. Most of this oxygen-depleted blood goes from the left ventricle into the aorta and on to the body. This anomaly requires surgical management to allow proper distribution of oxygen to the body.

## VASCULAR ANOMALIES

Vascular anomalies (noncardiac) are among the most common malformations in VCFS, reported by Shprintzen et al. (1997) as occurring in 100% of their series of cases. Vascular anomalies have been noted in the brain, thorax, limbs, and neck, with particularly unusual abnormalities of the carotid arteries resulting in concerns over surgery in the pharynx. These anomalies include:

65. Medially displaced and/or ectopic internal carotid arteries

66. Tortuous or kinked internal carotids

67. Jugular vein anomalies

68. Absence of internal carotid artery (unilateral)

69. Absence of vertebral artery (unilateral)

70. Tortuous or kinked vertebral arteries

71. Low bifurcation of common carotid

72. Reynaud's phenomenon

73. Small veins

74. Circle of Willis anomalies

### Medially Displaced and/or Ectopic Internal Carotid Arteries

The vascular anomaly that has received the greatest amount of attention in VCFS is abnormal placement and course of the internal carotid arteries in relation to the pharynx. First reported in 1987 in a clinical series of three cases, prominent pulsations of the internal carotid were seen during nasopharyngoscopy and confirmed as abnormal course and position using three-dimensional CT scans (MacKenzie-Stepner et al., 1987). Specifically, the arteries were found to be medially displaced in the pharynx at the level of the posterior pharyngeal wall and ectopic, meaning that they were close to the mucosal surface (Figure 2–37). The authors concluded that this placement would place the arteries directly in the surgical field for pharyngeal flap, risking severing of the major blood supply to the brain. In a prospective study of a consecutive series of individuals with VCFS using magnetic resonance angiography (MRA), it was found that endoscopic observations did not correlate well with the actual placement of the arteries (Mitnick, Bello, Golding-Kushner, Argamaso, & Shprintzen, 1996). In the series of 20 subjects, anomalies of the major neck vessels including the internal carotids were found in all cases, and

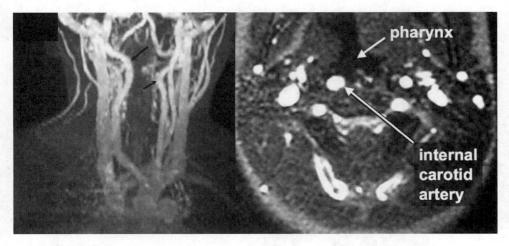

**FIGURE 2–37.** Ectopic, medially displaced internal carotid arteries.

in two cases (10% of the sample) the arteries were directly under the mucous membrane close to the midline of the pharynx at the base of the first cervical vertebra. The authors concluded that MRA should be performed prior to pharyngeal flap surgery. This recommendation was subsequently repeated by Tatum et al. (2002) in another series of 20 consecutive cases with similar findings from MRA.

## Tortuous or Kinked Internal Carotids

In addition to abnormal placement of the internal carotids, the arteries are often twisted, looped, or kinked (Figure 2–38). It is not clear if these anomalies expose patients with VCFS to any risk, such as stroke or occlusion of the arteries. The findings reported in VCFS and seen on MRA have been based on data from young children (Mitnick et al., 1996; Tatum, Chang, Havkin, & Shprintzen, 2002). Similar configurations of these arteries are found in the geriatric population, but not in children. The specific meaning of this coincidence is unclear but may be a fruitful area of research in the future.

## Jugular Vein Anomalies

Kinked and tortuous jugular veins and anomalous course of the jugular have also been noted in VCFS. There has not been an observed correlation between those cases where the carotids are anomalous and the jugular veins have had similar malformations.

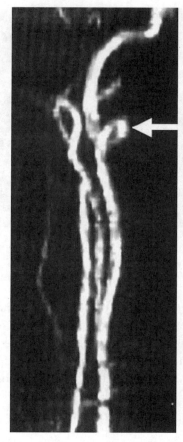

internal carotid artery
cervical loop

**FIGURE 2–38.** Tortuous internal carotid arteries.

## Absence of Internal Carotid Artery

A number of cases have been seen where the internal carotid disappears on MRA so that this major artery is either severely hypoplastic or aplastic (Mitnick et al., 1996). The A1 segment of the circle of Willis is absent in these cases, resulting in an obvious disturbance of the brain vasculature.

## Absence of Vertebral Artery

The vertebral artery is another of the major arteries that supplies blood to the brain. Absence of one branch of the vertebral artery has also been noted (Figure 2–39). Coexisting anomalies of the brain's vasculature have not been reported or studied to date.

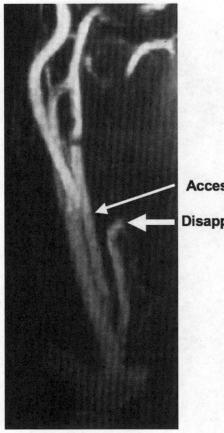

**FIGURE 2–39.** Absence of the vertebral artery in VCFS.

### Tortuous or Kinked Vertebral Arteries

Similar to the internal carotid arteries, the vertebral arteries may be tortuous or kinked in the majority of patients with VCFS (Figure 2-40). In our clinical sample of more than 120 MRAs, tortuosity of the vertebral artery was the most common vascular anomaly of the major neck vessels. In all cases studied to date, MRAs have been done on only one occasion. It is therefore not known if this tortuosity changes with age or if the tortuosity of these vessels is associated with any specific behavioral or cognitive impairments.

### Low Bifurcation of Common Carotid

The common carotid artery typically bifurcates to form the internal and external carotid arteries in the neck between C5 and C3. In VCFS, the bifurcation

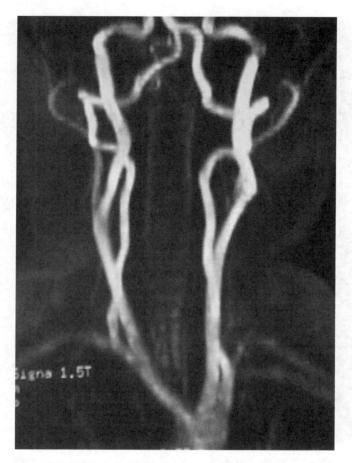

**FIGURE 2–40.** Tortuous vertebral arteries.

of the common carotid is often low, and in many cases occurs in the chest at the level of T1 to T3. Although this has no clinical significance in terms of perfusion to the brain, it does show that there is some type of primary malformation process affecting the carotid arteries and the blood supply to the brain. Because brain anomalies are a well-known feature of VCFS (as will be discussed later), one must wonder if the anomalies of the brain are related solely to genes that affect brain development, or if the problem is one of abnormal blood supply to the entire brain or parts of the brain, resulting in maldevelopment secondary to lack of perfusion (Shprintzen et al., 1997).

### Reynaud's Phenomenon

Reynaud's phenomenon is a relatively common vascular response to cold or sudden emotional distress. The small blood vessels in the peripheral parts of the body, typically the tips of the fingers and toes and on occasion the ears, the tip of the nose, and the lips, constrict, thereby trapping blood. The result is that the affected parts turn blue, and then bright red, and they may feel tingly or numb. In the general population, Reynaud's phenomenon does not typically occur until after puberty or later in life. In VCFS, Reynaud's phenomenon is seen even in newborns, infants, and young children. Other than the discomfort that is occasionally associated with Reynaud's phenomenon, there is no danger in its presence, but it may have diagnostic value in cases where VCFS has not yet been identified.

## Small Veins

Although there have been no comprehensive studies designed to measure blood vessels throughout the body in VCFS, there is clinical evidence that people with VCFS have smaller caliber veins. This has been observed when drawing blood from children with VCFS. Venipuncture is necessary to obtain blood for many of the necessary laboratory tests in VCFS, such as FISH, thyroid function tests, serum calcium levels, platelet analyses, and more. Because these children often require surgery on several occasions in their lives, it is necessary to establish lines to provide fluids and medications. In addition, the many research studies we have implemented over the years for genomic investigations have required venipuncture. The experience has shown us that it is very difficult to find large enough veins for obtaining sufficient blood to complete the tests. Although it is possible that these veins also collapse easily or constrict in response to the stick with the needle, we have found that finding sufficiently large vessels is problematic and the veins that are found are often in locations not commonly found in children.

## Circle of Willis Anomalies

The circle of Willis (Figure 2–41) is a complex of blood vessels at the base of the brain that forms a circle composed of a number of arterial segments. The circle of Willis receives blood from the internal carotid arteries and the basilar artery, which is formed by the joining of the vertebral arteries from each side of the neck. This blood is then distributed to the arteries that supply the brain. In VCFS, the circle of Willis is often abnormal and missing one or more segments (Figure 2–42). It is not known if abnormalities of the circle of Willis cause decreased blood flow to the brain or if lack of normal blood supply can result in embryonic brain growth failure, but this may be at least in part a viable explanation for some of the observations of brain anomalies in VCFS.

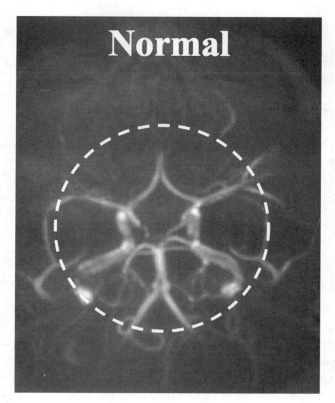

**FIGURE 2–41.** Normal circle of Willis.

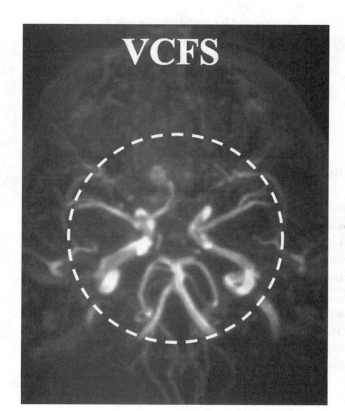

**FIGURE 2–42.** Abnormal circle of Willis in VCFS.

## BRAIN AND CENTRAL NERVOUS SYSTEM ANOMALIES

A number of researchers have been studying the brain in individuals with VCFS in great detail. The earliest reports on VCFS neuroanatomy were either anecdotal cases or clinical series (D. H. Altman, N. R. Altman, Mitnick, & Shprintzen, 1994; Lynch et al., 1996; Mitnick et al., 1994). Researchers then began to apply quantitative MR imaging of the brain to determine if specific areas of the brain might be deficient compared to nondeleted individuals. There is a high frequency of cavum septum pellucidum (Figure 2–43), a midline developmental anomaly of the brain, and we have observed asymmetric ventricular enlargement (Figure 2–44). We have also seen several cases of porencephalic cysts in our patients. More subtle anomalies observed on MRI studies have included cysts (Figure 2–45) and white matter hyperintensities (Figure 2–46) (Altman et al., 1994; Mitnick et al., 1994). These anomalies are

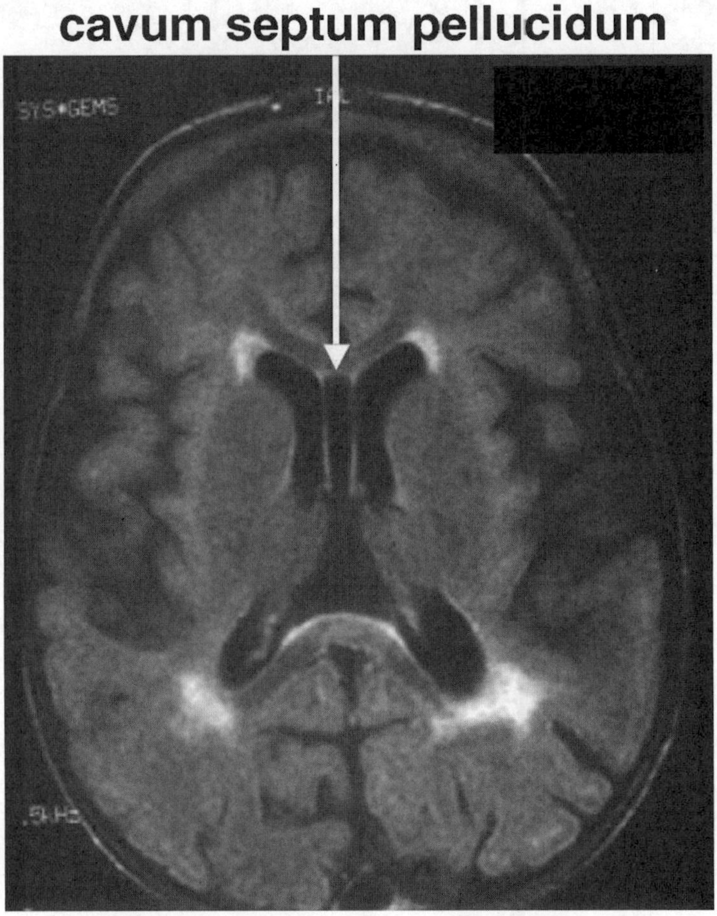

**FIGURE 2–43.** Cavum septum pellucidum in VCFS.

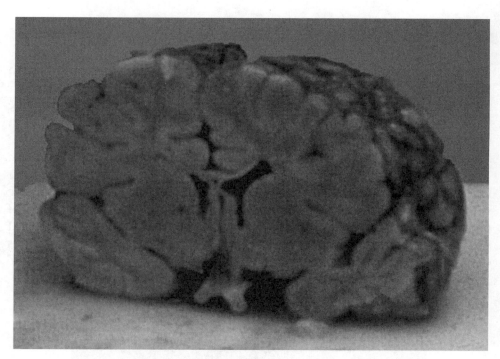

**FIGURE 2–44.** Asymmetric ventricles in VCFS.

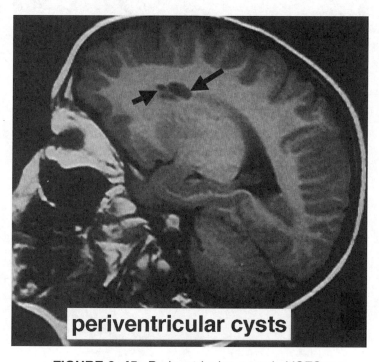

periventricular cysts

**FIGURE 2–45.** Periventricular cysts in VCFS.

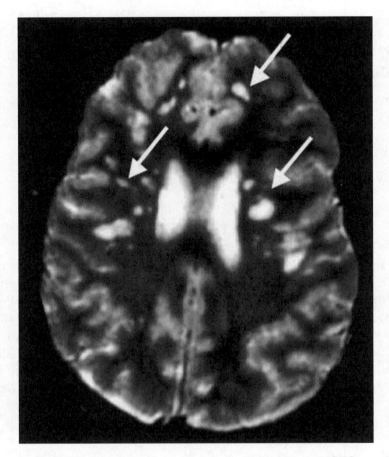

**FIGURE 2–46.** White matter hyperintensities in VCFS.

clearly related to errors in embryonic development, and research continues in an effort to find out the specific genes responsible for the anomalies. Brain and CNS anomalies include:

75. Reduced total brain volume

76. Variations in size of various brain segments, small cerebellar vermis and cerebellar hypoplasia

77. Periventricular cysts

78. White matter hyperintensities

79. Generalized hypotonia

80. Cerebellar ataxia

81. Seizures

82. Strokes

83. Spina bifida/meningomyelocele

84. Mild developmental delay

85. Enlarged Sylvian fissure

86. Cavum septum pellucidum

87. Pachygyria and polymicrogyria

88. Cortical dysgenesis or dysplasia

89. Arnold-Chiari anomaly

## Reduced Total Brain Volume

Several studies have demonstrated that the total brain volume in children with VCFS is reduced compared to normals and that the pattern of white matter distribution is different than normal (Barnea-Goraly et al., 2003; Chow, Zipursky, Mikulis, & Bassett, 2002; Eliez, Schmitt, White, & Reiss, 2000; Kates et al., 2006). This coincides with a higher prevalence of microcephaly in VCFS than in the general population. Research continues to be done assessing both whole brain volumes and the size of specific brain regions with the hope of correlating the type of variation in brain size with specific behavioral and learning features in the syndrome. At this point in time, no specific data of this type is available.

## Variations in Size of Various Brain Segments, Small Cerebellar Vermis, and Cerebellar Hypoplasia

A number of studies have shown specific variations in the volumes of specific brain regions including the reduced cerebellar volumes, reduced hippocampus volumes, reduced orbitofrontal cortex volumes, reduced prefrontal cortex volumes, increased amygdala volumes, and increased volumes of the corpus callosum (Debbane, Schaer, Farhoumand, Glaser, & Eliez, 2006; Kates, Antshel, Wilhite, Bessette, Abdul-Sabur, & Higgins, 2005; Kates et al., 2006; Shashi et al., 2004). Other studies have shown smaller cerebellar volumes (Chow et al., 1999; Devriendt, Thienen, Swillen, & Fryns, 1996; Eliez et al., 2000; Eliez et al., 2001; Lynch et al., 1995; Mitnick et al., 1994; van Amelsvoort, K. C. Murphy, & D. G. Murphy, 2001). Although hypotheses have been put forth to determine the effects of these variations, definitive links to brain volumes and behavior are still uncertain and are being studied in more detail with functional magnetic resonance studies. There may also be a link between motor development and cerebellar anomalies, but some recent studies have suggested a connection between the cerebellum and mental illness.

### Periventricular Cysts

Clinical and research MR studies have identified a number of variations in brain anatomy that occur with relatively high frequency in people with VCFS. One of these anomalies is the presence of small cysts, especially in the periventricular regions (Figure 2–47). No correlation has been made between the presence of these cysts and any particular neurologic, psychiatric, or cognitive pattern. The presumption is that these cysts represent some type of unspecified developmental anomaly. Although cysts of this type can be found in some normals, particularly of advanced age, they occur in more than one third of people with VCFS, therefore identifying them as a specific anomaly associated with the syndrome.

### White Matter Hyperintensities

White matter hyperintensities are named for their appearance in magnetic resonance imaging of the brain where they show up in the white matter of the cerebrum (Figure 2–48). They are also commonly called UBOs, an acronym for unidentified bright objects. More than one third of individuals with VCFS have this finding on MR imaging of the brain, although these hyperintensities are seen in normal people on rare occasion. As with periventricular cysts, the exact nature of these anomalies is unknown, and they do not appear to have

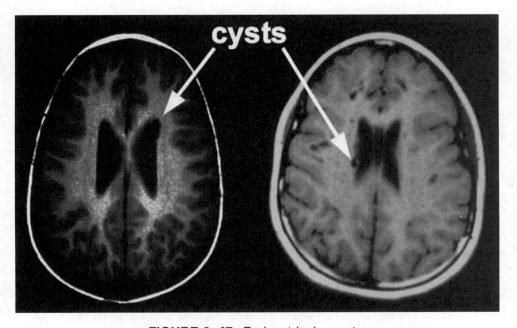

**FIGURE 2–47.** Periventricular cysts.

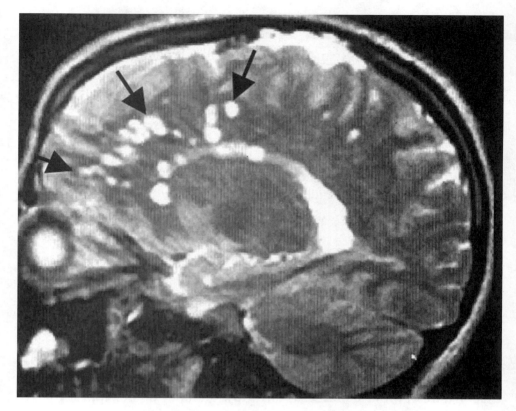

**FIGURE 2–48.** White matter hyperintensities (UBOs).

any specific relationship to mental or cognitive function. In the general population, UBOs are often seen in geriatric cases and are presumed to be related to demyelinization of the white matter tracts. UBOs are also found commonly in children with neurofibromatosis, type 1 (NF1), a syndrome that can also be associated with learning disabilities.

## Generalized Hypotonia

Hypotonia is a very common finding in VCFS and is clinically recognized in almost all cases. There are possibly two contributing factors to hypotonia in VCFS. It is typically presumed that hypotonia is related to central nervous system anomalies because so many syndromes with cognitive impairment have hypotonia as a clinical feature—disorders such as Down syndrome, Prader-Willi syndrome, X-linked mental retardation, Beckwith-Wiedemann syndrome, Smith-Lemli-Opitz syndrome, Cohen syndrome, Rett syndrome, Sotos syndrome, Wolf-Hirschhorn syndrome, and Kabuki syndrome to name just a few. However, hypotonia can also be caused by muscle weakness that is an anomaly of the muscle itself rather than the central nervous system's innervation of the muscles. There is some evidence for muscle abnormalities in VCFS that will be discussed later in relation to the pharyngeal and palatal muscle and evidence that the muscle fibers themselves are abnormal (Zim et al., 2003).

## Cerebellar Ataxia

Cerebellar ataxia has been reported in a single case of VCFS (Lynch et al., 1996) that was corroborated by abnormal cerebellar anatomy as seen on MR scanning. Movement disorders do occur in VCFS and, as with other components of the syndrome, may have multifactorial causes. Cerebellar involvement is always suspect because of the reported abnormalities associated with cerebellar structure (Chow et al., 1999; Devriendt et al., 1996; Eliez et al., 2000; Eliez et al., 2001; Lynch et al., 1995; Mitnick et al., 1994; van Amelsvoort et al., 2001), but it is also possible that dopamine regulation is abnormal because the gene that degrades dopamines, *COMT* (catechol-O-methyl-transferase), resides in the deleted region at 22q11.2. Dopamine, a neural transmitter, is essential to normal motor function and abnormalities of dopamine regulation can result in movement disorders; movement disorders in VCFS have been reported (Krahn, Maraganore, & Michels, 1998).

## Seizures

Another clinical finding in VCFS that has a complex or confusing etiology is seizures. Seizures in VCFS may be caused by hypocalcemia, high fevers, brain malformations, strokes, and abnormal electrical activity within the brain leading to epilepsy, with none of these being mutually exclusive. For example, high fevers are common in VCFS, especially during infancy and childhood, for those individuals who have immune deficiency or immune disorder. High fevers can lead to febrile seizures, but they can also lead to profuse sweating that depletes the body's calcium levels, causing a seizure. Individuals with VCFS, especially those who have had early heart surgery, may have had small strokes that could be asymptomatic until prompted by high fever or hypocalcemia. Seizures are actually more common in VCFS than might be expected, but the frequency of each type of seizure is not known. Reports of epileptiform activity in the brain have been published (Kao et al., 2004). Unprovoked seizures (not related to hypocalcemia, fever, or stroke) were reported to account for approximately 7% of all VCFS cases, with seizures of all types occurring in 16%. Shprintzen (1999) reported a higher frequency of seizures in VCFS, with 28% having at least one seizure, although the specific types of seizures were not reported and could not be determined. It is clear that seizures are a common, although not frequent, feature of VCFS and that isolating the cause of seizures may not be easy given the complexity and number of possible causes.

## Strokes

Strokes are another trait that could be caused by more than one anomaly. In some cases, particularly in infancy, strokes can occur after heart surgery. Clots from the surgery or dysfunctional heart valves and other structural anomalies of the heart and its vasculature can cause embolisms or thromboses that could block small brain vessels. It is also true, however, that individuals with VCFS have primary vascular anomalies including small caliber vessels, weak or thin vessel walls, and tortuous, twisted, or kinked vessels, all of which could cause abnormalities of blood flow resulting in strokes. Individuals with VCFS also have giant platelets that could potentially clog small and kinked vessels. As with other problems in VCFS, none of these are mutually exclusive. Although the period following cardiac surgery would be one of the times of highest risk for the occurrence of a stroke, they have been encountered later in life, and clinical experience has yielded several adolescents and young adults who had a sudden onset of seizures caused by strokes.

## Spina Bifida/Meningomyelocele

Several cases of meningomyeloceles with spina bifida have been reported in association with VCFS (Nickel & Magenis, 1996). It has been concluded that neural tube defects should be included among the anomalies caused by 22q11.2 deletions, a notion supported by the presence of both midline brain and spine malformations including holoprosencephaly and vertebral clefts (Ming et al., 1997; Wraith, Super, Watson, & Phillips, 1985). Although it appears that severe manifestations of neural tube defects are not common in VCFS, they do occur at a much higher rate than expected by chance. It has been estimated that among children with neural tube defects involving the spine who also have congenital heart anomalies and other clinical features that overlap with VCFS, nearly 20% may have 22q11.2 deletions (Nickel & Magenis, 1996). Therefore, although meningomyelocele may be an uncommon finding among children with VCFS, it may be more commonly found among children with neural tube defects than other multiple anomaly syndromes.

## Mild Developmental Delay

The majority of children with VCFS have a mild delay in the acquisition of motor milestones, or their development is at the outer range of normal. The average age of first independent steps in VCFS is 17 months, and less than a third of affected children walk before 15 months of age (Golding-Kushner, Weller, & Shprintzen, 1985). These borderline values are consistent with most other motor milestones and are also consistent with overall cognitive development patterns in the syndrome later in life. Speech onset is slightly more delayed, with first words typically being recognized at 19 months (Shprintzen, 2005b). It is possible that the more significant delay in speech onset is related to intelligibility issues centering on the presence of severe velopharyngeal insufficiency, but delays in language acquisition have also been reported (Scherer, D'Antonio, & Kalbfleisch, 1999). It is uniformly observed that expressive language is much more severely delayed than receptive language, but to date, no studies have focused on how the receptive impairment relates to the severe intelligibility problems encountered in VCFS. The mild delay of motor milestones may be related at least in part to the hypotonia described above.

### Enlarged Sylvian Fissure

The Sylvian fissure, also known as the lateral sulcus, separates the temporal lobe that sits below it from the parietal and frontal lobes that sit above it. The Sylvian fissure is one of the first landmarks of the brain to become noticeable in the embryonic period at approximately 14 weeks post-fertilization. A report of two cases with an enlarged Sylvian fissure was published in 1997 (Bingham et al., 1997), but this anomaly of a major brain landmark has not proven to be a common finding in the syndrome and may simply be another sign of an abnormal developmental process of the brain in people with VCFS that includes reduced total brain volume, smaller amygdala, smaller cerebellum, and cavum septum pellucidum.

### Cavum Septum Pellucidum

The septum pellucidum is a midline structure of the brain formed from two thin layers of glial tissue that typically fuses before or shortly after birth, creating a single plate of tissue that separates the lateral ventricles. If the two plates, or laminae, do not fuse, a fluid-filled region forms in the midline resulting in a cavum septum pellucidum (Figure 2–49). A cavum septum pellucidum present at birth closes in more than 80% of individuals so that it is not typically present after the neonatal period. Because the glial tissue that makes up the septum pellucidum is contiguous with the limbic system of the brain, some researchers believe that cavum septum pellucidum may be associated with limbic system pathology. The limbic system mediates emotional responses and also plays a role in the formation of memory, both of which show some impairment in VCFS. Although cavum septum pellucidum is found in about 10% of normal people, it does occur in a higher percentage of people with schizophrenia (Galarza, Merlo, Ingratta, E. F. Albanese, & A. M. Albanese, 2004), perhaps as much as three times higher than in the general population. Cavum septum pellucidum occurs much more frequently in people with VCFS, in well over 90% of more than 250 cases receiving MR scans at Upstate Medical

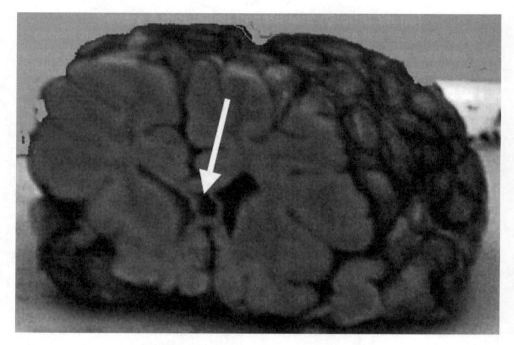

**FIGURE 2–49.** Cavum septum pellucidum.

University. It should be noted that the frequency of psychosis in VCFS is far higher than it is in the general population, but as all scientists understand, correlations do not firmly establish cause-and-effect relationships. The question is if the mental illness associated with VCFS is related to structural anomalies of the brain, is it signaled by the presence of cavum septum pellucidum.

## Pachygyria and Polymicrogyria

A small number of cases of pachygyria and polymicrogyria have been reported in association with VCFS (Ehara, Maegaki, & Takeshita, 2003; Koolen et al., 2004; Robin et al., 2006). It is unclear at this time if this significant brain malformation involving abnormal gyration of the cortex is a primary effect of the deletion or a problem associated with vascular supply to the brain (Shprintzen et al., 1997).

## Cortical Dysgenesis or Dysplasia

Several cases of cortical dysgenesis have been reported in the medical literature (Bird, 2001; Bird & Scambler, 2000). We have also seen several other cases, some with severe cortical abnormalities and profound developmental impairment, including one case with near total cortical agenesis. This severe malformation of the brain could also potentially be related to vascular anomalies or even severe oxygen deprivation to the brain.

### Arnold-Chiari Anomaly

The frequency of Arnold-Chiari anomaly (sometimes simply called Chiari malformation or ACM) in VCFS is not known, but this problem associated with the herniation of the cerebellar tonsils into and through the foramen magnum has been observed in multiple cases of VCFS. Although many people, with or without VCFS, may have Arnold-Chiari anomaly that is asymptomatic and therefore never clinically detected, in some cases there can be compression of the cerebellum, brainstem, and cranial nerves with obstruction of flow of cerebrospinal fluid. Symptoms can include dizziness, syncope, muscle weakness, numbness, double vision, headache, and balance or coordination problems. When symptomatic, surgical management is possible.

## PHARYNGEAL, LARYNGEAL, AND AIRWAY ANOMALIES

The pharynx and larynx are anomalous in a high percentage of individuals with VCFS (Chegar et al., 2006; Shprintzen, 2005b). Structural asymmetry of one or more parts of the airway was found in approximately 70% of subjects with VCFS by Chegar et al. (2006) and absence or hypoplasia of the adenoid was found in more than 80% of individuals with VCFS by Williams et al. (1987). Because many individuals with VCFS require surgery in the pharynx, understanding the anomalies associated with respiratory, speech, and feeding difficulties becomes very important. Upper airway anomalies include:

90. Upper airway obstruction in infancy

91. Absent or small adenoids, large palatine tonsils

92. Laryngeal web (anterior)

93. Large pharyngeal airway

94. Laryngomalacia

95. Arytenoid/corniculate hyperplasia

96. Pharyngeal hypotonia

97. Thin pharyngeal muscle

98. Asymmetric pharyngeal movement

99. Structurally asymmetric pharynx

100. Unilateral vocal cord paresis

101. Structurally asymmetric larynx

102. Reactive airway disease/asthma

## Upper Airway Obstruction in Infancy

Respiratory or feeding difficulty secondary to upper airway obstruction in infancy are common in VCFS. Documented obstructive apnea has been found in 23% of neonates and infants with VCFS and failure-to-thrive in 74% (Shprintzen, 1999). The most common cause of early feeding difficulties in infants is upper airway compromise, and this combination is common in VCFS (Shprintzen, 2005b). As with other functional problems in VCFS, upper airway obstruction is also multifactorial in etiology. Factors that can contribute to airway obstruction include laryngomalacia, laryngeal web, hypotonia, retrognathia, tonsillar hypertrophy, vocal cord paralysis, vascular anomalies in the chest that might induce negative pressure in the upper airway by constricting the trachea, increasing respiratory effort, and extraesophageal reflux. As is the case with other multifactorial traits, none of these problems is mutually exclusive. It is therefore critically important to have a thorough differential diagnosis that includes appropriate imaging procedures. Flexible fiberoptic nasopharyngolaryngoscopy is mandatory. Bronchoscopy and MR imaging may also be necessary.

## Absent or Small Adenoids, Large Palatine Tonsils

Williams et al. (1987) reported that the adenoid was small or absent in more than 80% of individuals with VCFS. Because the adenoid pad is the primary site of contact for the velum against the posterior aspect of the pharynx in normal children (Video 2–8), the absence or hypoplasia of the adenoid places children with VCFS at risk for developing velopharyngeal insufficiency (VPI), especially with other factors affecting the function of the velopharynx possibly coexisting with adenoid abnormalities (Havkin, Tatum, & Shprintzen, 2000). It is possible that a normal amount of adenoid tissue might appear smaller than normal in an enlarged pharynx with a deficient palate, both conditions commonly seen in VCFS. However, the complete absence of adenoid tissue in some cases of VCFS clearly implies a primary hypoplasia in the syndrome. Golding-Kushner (1991) found that adenoid size was smaller than normal in VCFS and, in addition, the adenoids occupied a significantly smaller proportion of the nasopharyngeal space than normal. Golding-Kushner (1991) also found that individuals with VCFS who had the largest velopharyngeal gaps during speech were those with the smallest adenoids. Havkin et al. (2000) found that the single most important predictor of which individuals with VCFS would develop VPI was adenoid size. Therefore, congenital absence or hypoplasia of the adenoid may be used as an early warning for the development of VPI and severe hypernasality, therefore emphasizing the need to develop strategies for preventing the development of compensatory articulation patterns in VCFS.

It should be noted that contrary to adenoid hypoplasia, the palatine tonsils in VCFS tend to be large and often require surgical removal. Hypertrophic tonsils are a frequent finding in VCFS (Shprintzen, 2000a). In some cases, hypertrophic tonsils can contribute to VPI by interfering with palatal or lateral pharyngeal wall motion (Shprintzen et al., 1987). The most common symptoms caused by tonsillar hypertrophy are feeding difficulties, sleep disordered breathing, chronic mouth-open posture, choking, coughing, and abnormal oral resonance. The tonsils are often seen approximating the epiglottis and the aryepiglottic folds, thus inducing a laryngeal adductor reflex and the coughing and choking symptoms (Video 2-9).

## Laryngeal Web (Anterior)

Anterior laryngeal webs (also known as glottic webs) are rare congenital malformations, but a high percentage if not the majority of people with laryngeal web have VCFS. In a consecutive series of 17 individuals with laryngeal web ascertained over 30 months in a busy otolaryngology program in Cincinnati, Miyamoto et al. (2004) reported that 11 of the cases had VCFS. Although laryngeal web is a low frequency anomaly in VCFS, probably occurring in less than 10% of cases (Shprintzen, 1999), it is possible that a major percentage of people with laryngeal web have VCFS. In most cases, the laryngeal webs found in VCFS are thin membranous anterior webs (Figure 2-50) that can be seen on fiberoptic endoscopy of the upper airway. When small, the webs can be asymptomatic in terms of respiration, yet cause hoarseness, high pitched voice, or mild inspiratory stridor or stertor that may be interpreted as laryngomalacia. More severe cases have been encountered, including subglottic webs and thicker fibrous webs (Figure 2-51). Although laryngeal web has not typically been a major treatment issue in the majority of cases with VCFS, it is certainly a strong diagnostic indicator for the syndrome. Any neonate with a laryngeal web should have FISH for a 22q11.2 deletion, and suspicion of the diagnosis of VCFS should increase significantly if congenital heart disease, facial asymmetry, hypotonia, or cleft palate is also present.

## Large Pharyngeal Airway

The frequency of hypernasal speech secondary to velopharyngeal insufficiency (VPI) in VCFS is very high (approximately 75% of cases). As will be discussed later in this chapter, the high frequency of VPI in VCFS has multiple causes, among them being a larger than normal pharyngeal volume (Golding-Kushner, 1991; Shprintzen, 1982). Pharyngeal volume is increased by a number of factors

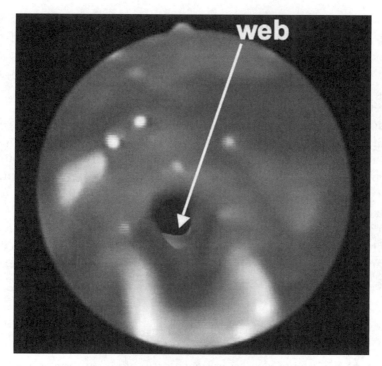

**FIGURE 2–50.** Thin membranous laryngeal web in VCFS. This web was asymptomatic.

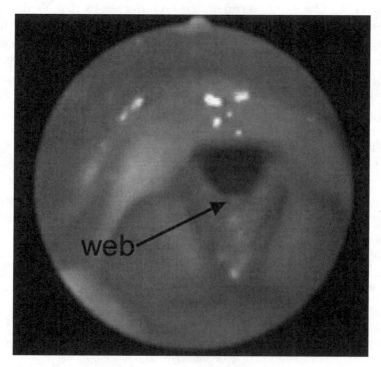

**FIGURE 2–51.** Thick fibrous laryngeal web in VCFS that was symptomatic for airway obstruction.

including the shortening of the palate that comes with overt or submucous clefting (Golding-Kushner, 1991; Shprintzen, 1982, 2000a, 2005a), smaller than normal adenoid mass (Williams et al., 1987), decreased muscle wall thickness (Golding-Kushner, 1991; Zim et al., 2003), and platybasia (Arvystas & Shprintzen, 1984; Golding-Kushner, 1991). The increased volume of the pharynx requires vigorous movement from the palate and pharyngeal walls in order to achieve velopharyngeal closure, but the opposite is true in VCFS, with documented hypotonia of the pharynx (Golding-Kushner, 1991; Zim et al., 2003) resulting in reduced movement of the pharyngeal and palatal musculature.

## Laryngomalacia

Laryngomalacia can be translated as "soft larynx" and typically refers to the cartilages of the larynx that are above the vocal cords collapsing during inspiration, causing a brief obstruction of the airway. Laryngomalacia is a common disorder of infancy and typically resolves with increasing age. When present in the neonatal period, laryngomalacia usually resolves without treatment by 6 months of age or shortly after as the airway enlarges and the cartilages become more firm. Many clinicians think of laryngomalacia as being isolated to the epiglottis, which can curl onto itself (Figure 2–52) with a resulting omega shape at rest (Figure 2–53). However, the arytenoids and corniculate cartilages can also collapse, causing laryngomalacia by falling in on the vocal cords and briefly obstructing the airway (Figure 2–54).

Laryngomalacia typically results in brief and not very severe oxygen desaturations, usually between 80 and 85%. This is because the collapse typically occurs at the very end of a breath as negative pressure is induced into the upper airway, causing the soft neonatal cartilages to be sucked in towards the vocal cords (Video 2–10). Treatment is not usually required to resolve laryngomalacia because the desaturations are so brief and most typically occur when the infant is awake and taking deeper breaths. Laryngomalacia is less severe during sleep when there is less negative pressure during respiration because of the slower respiratory rate and more shallow breaths. The best treatment is typically time, unless the obstructions are more severe with desaturations that consistently fall below 80% for more than several seconds. In VCFS, hypotonia is common and laryngomalacia may last more than the typical few months it is seen in the general population.

Diagnostic evidence of laryngomalacia includes high-pitched inspiratory squeaks at the end of breaths, brief desaturations without distress in the infant, and absence of cyanosis. The definitive diagnostic procedure for laryngomalacia is fiberoptic endoscopy of the upper airway with direct observation of the larynx during respiration. The symptoms of laryngomalacia (intermittent desaturation and respiratory noises) can also occur in a variety of other laryngeal or upper airway obstructions that might not have the same natural history as laryngomalacia.

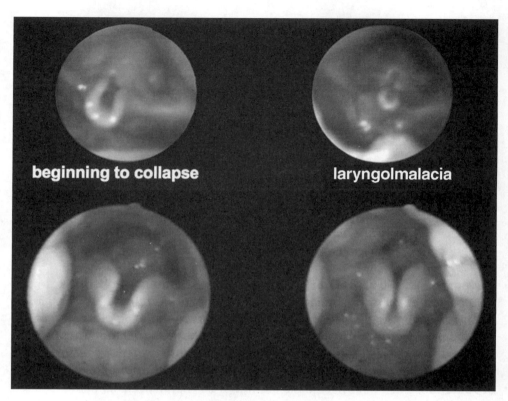

**FIGURE 2–52.** Laryngomalacia involving the epiglottis.

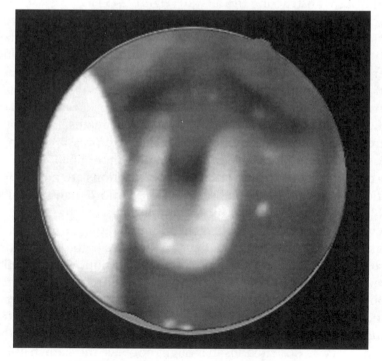

**FIGURE 2–53.** Omega-shaped epiglottis.

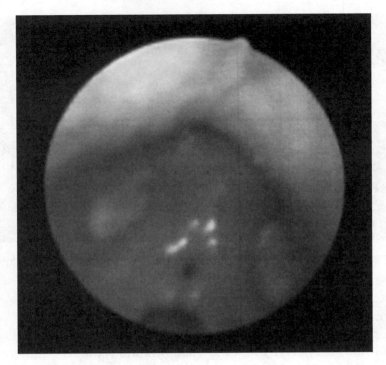

**FIGURE 2–54.** Laryngomalacia involving the arytenoids.

## Arytenoid/Corniculate Hyperplasia

Enlarged arytenoid and corniculate cartilages are often associated with chronic extraesophageal reflux that irritates the laryngeal structures. This type of irritation will cause edema of the mucosa covering the arytenoids and corniculate cartilages, but the cartilages themselves are not anomalous. In VCFS, we have observed a variety of anomalies of the arytenoids and surrounding structures, including asymmetry, abnormally long arytenoids and corniculates, and short aryepiglottic folds (Figure 2-55, Video 2-11). These anomalies have been found in individuals with no evidence of reflux or other irritations of the larynx.

## Pharyngeal Hypotonia

When we initially described pharyngeal hypotonia in VCFS (Shprintzen et al., 1978), the clinical feature was based on observations of the pharynx during speech that showed an absence of movement of the velum and pharyngeal walls in most cases. There are other possible explanations for this lack of movement, ranging from learning to the consistent observation that in the presence of compensatory articulation patterns, the velopharyngeal valve does not typically move even in individuals who do not have VCFS. It was not until

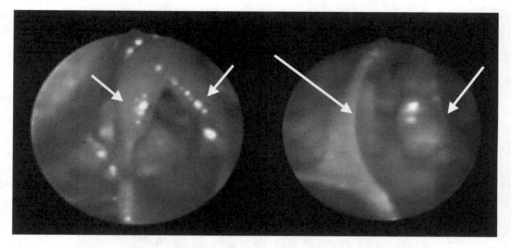

**FIGURE 2–55.** Anomalies of the arytenoids, corniculates, and aryepiglottic folds.

the histological study of Zim et al. (2003) that hard evidence was obtained showing muscle fiber anomalies in the pharynx that would result in reduced movement during speech. Zim et al. (2003) found reduced numbers of type 1 fibers in the superior constrictor muscles of individuals with VCFS, and the fibers that were present had smaller diameters than normal.

## Thin Pharyngeal Muscle

Zim et al. (2003) also found that the muscle wall of the pharynx in VCFS was thinner than normal, confirming an earlier study by Golding-Kushner (1991). The thinner muscle in VCFS can have surgical implications for reconstruction of the velopharyngeal valve, as would be done during pharyngeal flap surgery. Although thickness of the posterior pharyngeal wall has not been specifically correlated to degree of muscular movement in the pharynx as yet, the high frequency of reduced movement in VCFS accompanies a high frequency of absent movement in the pharyngeal walls.

## Asymmetric Pharyngeal Movement

Although lateral pharyngeal wall motion during speech is absent in a large number of individuals with VCFS who have hypernasal speech, in those cases where there is some lateral wall motion, asymmetric motion is seen in more than 60% of cases (Chegar et al., 2006). Asymmetric lateral pharyngeal wall motion also has implications for treatment of VPI and hypernasal speech (Argamaso, Levandowski, Golding-Kushner, & Shprintzen, 1994; Skolnick & McCall, 1972). Centrally placed pharyngeal flaps or sphincter pharyngoplasties are likely to fail because velopharyngeal gaps would be skewed to one side, requiring specifically placed flaps (Argamaso et al., 1994). Therefore, it is important for clinicians to be aware that asymmetric movement is common in VCFS, and that specific diagnosis of VPI by a combination of multiview videofluoroscopy and nasopharyngoscopy is critical to prescribing surgical management (Golding-Kushner et al., 1990).

## Structurally Asymmetric Pharynx

A recent and interesting finding in VCFS was reported by Chegar et al. (2006), who reviewed endoscopic and fluoroscopic data from 121 subjects with VCFS and compared them to similar data from a control sample of children who did not have VCFS. Structural asymmetry of the pharynx was found in more than three quarters of subjects with VCFS (Figure 2–56; Video 2–12)

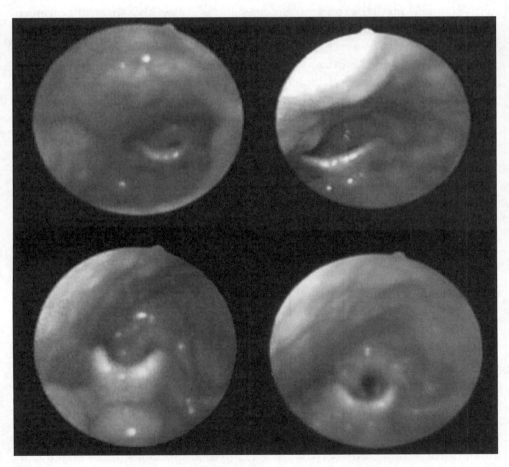

**FIGURE 2–56.** Asymmetry of the posterior pharyngeal wall in a series of four cases of VCFS.

but in few normal controls, resulting in a statistically significant difference (Chegar et al., 2006). There was a threefold preponderance of increased fullness on the right side of the pharynx compared to the left, and the lateral pharyngeal walls were also asymmetrically placed in relation to the midline in more than half of the cases reviewed using endoscopic and radiographic studies. The embryologic significance of these findings is not known, nor its basic genetic cause, as yet, but the pharyngeal findings are only one component in a series of asymmetries in the craniofacial complex and elsewhere in the body including the ears, the kidneys, and the face.

## Unilateral Vocal Cord Paresis

In children with congenital heart disease, it has often been observed that there is unilateral vocal cord paresis following heart surgery. It is common for patients to receive explanations that this asymmetry of vocal cord movement with reduced medial excursion on one side is caused by surgical complications, often postulated to be damage to the recurrent laryngeal nerve. In almost all cases, this type of nerve damage is supposed, not confirmed. It is possible that in many cases of cardiac surgery in infants that result in observed vocal cord paresis, the patients actually had VCFS. The vocal cord paresis seen in VCFS is congenital and not traumatically induced. In our own series of cases, the frequency of vocal cord paresis is no different in those cases with or without heart anomalies and cardiothoracic surgery (Chegar et al., 2006). Although true vocal cord paralysis is seen in VCFS, partial paresis is far more common (Video 2-13). In rare cases, unilateral vocal cord paralysis is seen, and even more rarely, bilateral vocal cord paralysis, but the majority of cases represent reduced movement in one cord, and it is most often the left cord, although right-sided cases are also found. Symptomatically, hoarse voice and high-pitched voice are common in VCFS as will be discussed later, but although it can be hypothesized that these symptoms are related to structural and functional laryngeal anomalies, this cannot be conclusively confirmed as yet.

## Structurally Asymmetric Larynx

Asymmetric laryngeal structure, including asymmetry of the vocal cords (Figure 2-57), asymmetry of the epiglottis (Figure 2-58), and asymmetry of the arytenoids and corniculates (Figure 2-59) have all been observed and reported in VCFS (Chegar et al., 2006). Differences in the size of the vibrating mass of the vocal cords certainly result in voice problems, most specifically hoarseness, but the asymmetry of the epiglottis and arytenoids is probably asymptomatic in most cases.

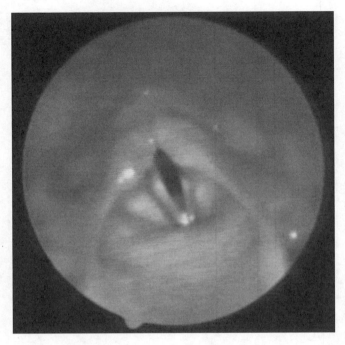

**FIGURE 2–57.** Asymmetric vocal cord thickness in VCFS.

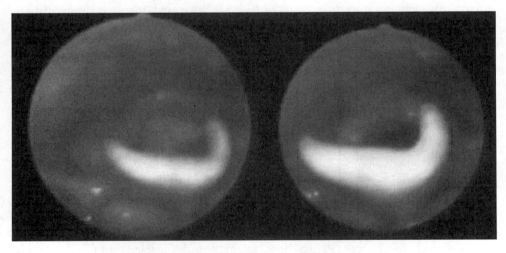

**FIGURE 2–58.** Asymmetric epiglottis in VCFS.

## Reactive Airway Disease/Asthma

Lower respiratory illness in VCFS can be both acute, as in pneumonia, bronchitis, and bronchiolitis, and chronic. The chronic lower respiratory illness in VCFS is often thought to be asthma, but in most cases the symptoms are more

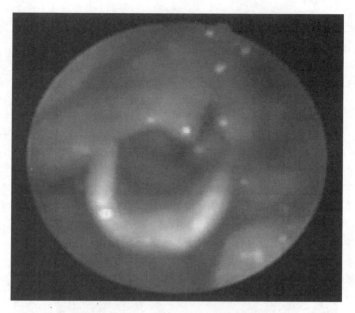

**FIGURE 2–59.** Asymmetric arytenoids and corniculates in VCFS.

consistent with a persistent reactive airway disease that becomes exacerbated during upper respiratory infections or periods of stress. Although the treatment for asthma and reactive airway disease are essentially the same, recognizing the problem as a chronic issue that is less likely to have the same sudden onsets as seen in asthma would be of importance.

## ABDOMINAL AND VISCERAL ANOMALIES

A variety of anomalies of the abdominal wall and internal organs have been observed in VCFS, some being very common. Inguinal hernias and diastasis recti are common congenital anomalies in humans, and umbilical hernias are so common among newborns that in some cases these are considered to be variants of normal because they spontaneously close within weeks or months. The importance of recognizing these anomalies focuses less on the treatment and more on the diagnostic significance. Although common congenital malformations, if an inguinal hernia, umbilical hernia, or unilateral renal agenesis were to occur in association with congenital heart disease, cleft palate, nasal regurgitation, asymmetric crying facies, or Robin sequence, then FISH for VCFS is indicated unless another obvious diagnosis with the same findings is evident, such as Down syndrome.

Anomalies reported in VCFS involving the abdomen and internal organs include:

103. Hypoplastic/aplastic kidney

104. Cystic kidneys

105. Inguinal hernias

106. Umbilical hernias

107. Diastasis recti

108. Diaphragmatic hernia

109. Malrotation of bowel

110. Hepatoblastoma and other tumors

## Hypoplastic/Aplastic and Cystic or Horseshoe Kidneys

Unilateral agenesis or hypoplasia of the kidneys is a relatively common anomaly in VCFS, and cystic or horseshoe kidneys are somewhat less frequent, but renal anomalies are reported at a frequency of approximately 21% (Shprintzen, 1999). This may be an underestimate because unilateral absence of a kidney or a smaller than normal kidney is a silent anomaly and therefore undetected in many cases unless renal ultrasounds are specifically ordered. Whenever the diagnosis of VCFS is made, renal ultrasounds should be done to determine renal anatomy. Although treatment is rarely necessary, the knowledge of unilateral renal agenesis is potentially important. In some cases, bilateral renal agenesis may occur, but this will be discussed in relation to Potter sequence later in this chapter. The mechanism for the absence of one or both kidneys is not understood at present. It is possible that one of the deleted genes participates in formation of the renal system so that hemizygosity of that gene causes hypoplasia or aplasia. However, this would not really explain unilateral aplasia, with the remaining kidney being normal. A second hypothesis that may be responsible for many developmental anomalies in VCFS is that there is absence of the vascular supply to the developing kidney, so that it never fully develops. We actually have anecdotal evidence of this in a single autopsy of a baby with VCFS showing unilateral aplasia of the kidney with unusual cystic remnants of some tissue in that location and absence of the renal artery on that side (Figure 2–60).

## Inguinal Hernias

Inguinal hernias may be unilateral or bilateral in VCFS, and are often associated with hypospadias in males. Inguinal hernias typically require surgical repair because they run the risk of a bowel entrapment if not corrected. There is no contraindication to surgical correction unless the cardiac status of the child prevents any major surgical intervention.

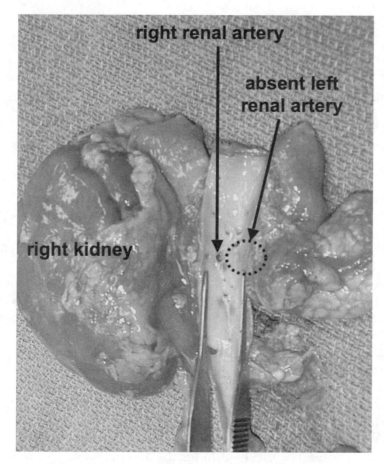

**FIGURE 2–60.** Unilateral absence of the kidney in a baby with VCFS that did not survive infancy. Note the absence of the renal artery on that side with the presence of cystlike and dysplastic tissues on that side.

## Umbilical Hernias

Umbilical hernias (Figure 2-61) are very common in the general population and, when they are small, rarely require treatment and do not present as health risks to children. In rare cases if they are very large, surgical correction may be needed, or elective surgery may be requested for esthetic reasons. Umbilical hernias occur in nearly 40% of children with VCFS (Shprintzen, 1999), a much larger number than would be expected in the general population.

## Diastasis Recti

Diastasis recti is a separation of muscular wall of the abdomen above the level of the umbilicus. Diastasis recti occurs in more than 20% of individuals with

VCFS and is seen in higher frequency among cases with umbilical hernia. In some cases, there is a somewhat atypical diastasis recti with the hernia being isolated to a small circular area or even off-center (Figure 2–62). In most cases, surgical repair of these defects is unnecessary, and because the defects are higher on the abdomen than the umbilicus or any natural creases in the skin, surgery leaves behind a scar that may be as esthetically objectionable as the actual hernia.

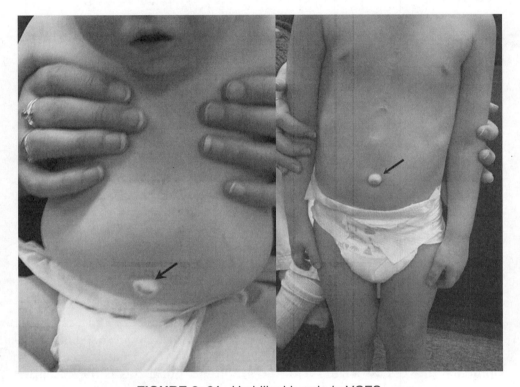

**FIGURE 2–61.** Umbilical hernia in VCFS.

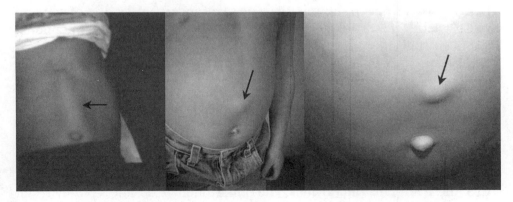

**FIGURE 2–62.** Diastasis recti, including atypical cases, in VCFS.

## Diaphragmatic Hernia

Diaphragmatic hernias can be serious anomalies because defects in the diaphragm will allow the intestines to push into the thoracic cavity causing compression of the lung and in some cases the heart, resulting in hypoventilation, tachypnea, and tachycardia. As is true in infants without VCFS who have diaphragmatic hernia, the majority of these defects in VCFS are left-sided. Diaphragmatic hernia typically requires immediate surgical correction because the respiratory and cardiac symptoms are life-threatening.

## Malrotation of Bowel

Malrotation of the gut is a twisting of the intestine that is rare in VCFS but does occur at a higher frequency than as an isolated anomaly in the general population. Not all malrotations are symptomatic, but in the majority of cases the twisting causes a partial or complete obstruction of the bowel, necessitating surgical correction. Because children with VCFS are typically constipated (discussed in more detail later in this chapter), milder malrotations may go undiagnosed. In cases of severe constipation, malrotation should be suspected in VCFS and ruled out.

## Hepatoblastoma and Other Tumors

Several children with VCFS have been found to have rare malignant tumors, including hepatoblastoma. The significance of these cancers in a very small sample of children with VCFS is unknown. Blastomas are comprised of immature undifferentiated embryonic cells and may represent an abnormal developmental process associated with the syndrome, but if this is the case, the event is extremely rare, and is certainly less than 1% of all cases. It is also possible that genes in the deleted region play a role in tumor suppression and the deletion may, in rare cases, prevent the suppression of embryonic tumors. There is no evidence to show at this time that cancers are a cause of concern in VCFS, and to date, the few cases that have been encountered in children have been congenital.

# LIMB ANOMALIES

The large majority of limb anomalies in VCFS are minor or even variants of normal. Although there are occasional major limb anomalies associated with VCFS, these are rare and obvious. The minor findings do not typically result in any functional problems and therefore are primarily of diagnostic significance. The limb anomalies associated with VCFS include:

111. Small hands and feet

112. Tapered digits

113. Short fingernails

114. Rough, red, scaly skin on hands and feet, morphea

115. Contractures

116. Triphalangeal thumbs

117. Polydactyly

118. Soft tissue syndactyly

### Small Hands and Feet

The majority of individuals with VCFS have small hands and feet, although many clinicians mistakenly believe that the fingers are long. Although long fingers have been seen in a small number of individuals with VCFS, the majority of people with VCFS have small hands and short fingers, but the fingers are proportionate to palmar length. The feet also are small. It should be anticipated that the most peripheral portion of the limbs would be small in VCFS because of poor peripheral perfusion. Although the growth of major blood vessels is genetically determined, in the periphery, the major driving force for growth is perfusion through the small vessels. People with severe heart disease tend to have blunted fingertips because the force of perfusion to the most distal parts of the body is reduced.

### Tapered Digits

Tapering of the digits so that the fingertips are narrower than the middle phalanges and base of the fingers is very common in VCFS (Figure 2–63). Tapering of the fingertips may be a primary gene effect, but it is far more likely to be secondary to decreased peripheral perfusion.

### Short Fingernails

Fingernails also depend on peripheral perfusion for growth because the length of the nail bed is linked to the length of the distal phalanges of the fingers. In general, the nail on each digit occupies at least half of the distance from the

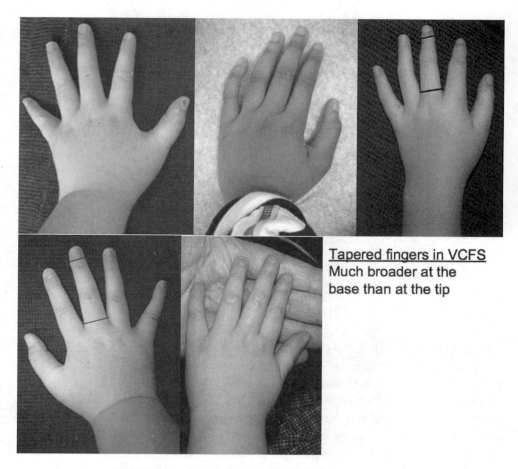

Tapered fingers in VCFS
Much broader at the
base than at the tip

**FIGURE 2–63.** Tapering of the fingers in VCFS.

distal joint to the tip of the finger (Figure 2-64). In individuals with VCFS, the nail is much shorter (Figure 2-64) and blunted, typically for all digits, but occasionally for several fingers.

## Rough, Red, Scaly Skin on Hands and Feet, Morphea

Also consistent with reduced perfusion is the development of rough, scaly skin on the palms and soles of the feet. It is also possible that this may be a type of autoimmune response consistent with other autoimmune disorders found in VCFS, such as thyroiditis and juvenile rheumatoid arthritis. However, autoimmune problems in VCFS are not very common, whereas circulatory problems are. In more severe cases, the rough skin on the hands is invaded by fibrous tissue causing the skin to lose its elasticity, a condition known as morphea.

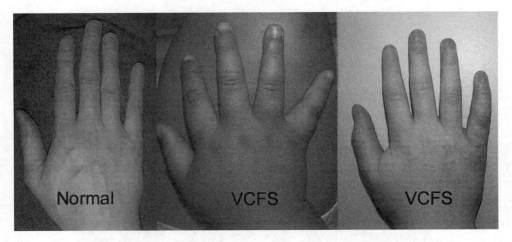

**FIGURE 2–64.** Normal fingernail length (*left*) compared to the typical length of the nail in VCFS (*center and right*).

## Contractures

In the most severe cases of skin changes, the skin loses so much elasticity that the fingers are unable to straighten, resulting in joint contractures of the fingers. Contractures of larger joints have not been reported in VCFS, and it is therefore likely that this problem, although extremely rare in VCFS, is caused by poor circulation.

## Triphalangeal Thumbs

The thumbs are the only digits in humans that have two bones (phalanges), while the remaining eight digits have three. However, some individuals with VCFS have been reported to have three phalanges, a condition that can also be associated with a number of other multiple anomaly syndromes. It is known that disturbance of perfusion to the developing limb buds can cause a variety of anomalies of the hands and fingers, including triphalangeal thumbs, so a variety of finger anomalies is not unexpected in VCFS.

## Polydactyly

Polydactyly, usually post-axial, occurs in a small percentage of individuals with VCFS, probably less than 5% of patients, but it does occur at a frequency higher than seen in the general population. In most cases, the extra digit is a small, incompletely formed finger or a small nubbin adjacent to the fifth finger (Figure 2-65). These extra digits are typically removed in infancy.

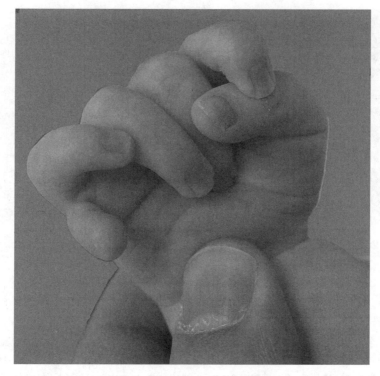

**FIGURE 2–65.** Post-axial polydactyly in patients with VCFS.

## Soft Tissue Syndactyly

Mild soft tissue syndactyly is another uncommon finding in VCFS that can be related to poor embryonic peripheral perfusion. The syndactyly is typically between the second and third fingers or toes, but occurs in a very small number of cases and typically does not require treatment.

## PROBLEMS IN INFANCY

Infancy is a difficult time for many babies with VCFS. Besides congenital heart disease, which is the major threat to life, feeding difficulties and general discomfort and malaise caused by a variety of problems often result in family stress and unhappiness in the baby and the family. Moreover, these early findings are highly suggestive of the diagnosis of VCFS even when congenital heart disease is not present and should raise suspicions sufficiently to warrant FISH studies. Common problems in the neonatal period, infancy, and toddler years include:

119.  Feeding difficulty

120.  Failure-to-thrive

121.  Chronic constipation

122.  Gastroesophageal reflux (GER or GERD)

123.  Nasal regurgitation

124.  Irritability

## Feeding Difficulty

As has been true with many other anomalies described previously, feeding difficulties in VCFS are complicated and multifactorial in etiology. There are very few reports in the literature analyzing feeding problems, and those that have been published are anecdotal reports without controlled analysis of findings (Eicher et al., 2000; Rommel et al., 1999). The focus has been on abnormalities of the end-organ (the pharynx and esophagus) without substantive evidence that any functional abnormalities of these structures exist in VCFS when compared to normals.

Feeding in VCFS can be affected by airway compromise, hypotonia, structural anomalies of the palate and pharynx, vascular anomalies that can impinge on the esophagus, slow gastric emptying, chronic constipation, irritable temperament, overall constitutional weakness secondary to congenital heart disease and other health issues, and surgical procedures.

### Airway Compromise

The majority of feeding disorders in infants are related to some type of airway compromise. As discussed earlier, airway disorders in VCFS may be of either the upper airway or the lower airway, or both. Robin sequence, hypotonia, abnormal vascular compression of the trachea, pulmonary valve or artery anomalies, and hypertrophic tonsils can all cause airway compromise singly or together. Because the pharynx is both the entry to the larynx and the esophagus, both food and air must pass through it, sometimes at the same time. When there are problems with airflow through the pharynx, especially during eating when the presence of a bolus of food may contribute to that compromise, babies will always opt for breathing over eating. Before looking for explanations relating to pharyngeal or esophageal movements, the clinician should always look towards the airway first as a potential source of feeding problems. Even if the airway is marginally functional, if it is difficult for the baby to breathe while eating, much more energy will be expended in the feeding process, therefore tiring more rapidly during feeding and becoming more irritable (Video 2–14). Rather than a normal suck-swallow-breathe pattern, airway compromise causes the baby to breathe more often and more forcefully to maintain proper oxygen saturation. The more effort the baby expends, the more calories are burned and the less weight gain. It is therefore essential in such cases to identify the source of the airway obstruction and relieve it or find a way to accommodate better feeding in a shorter period of time.

### Hypotonia

Hypotonia can contribute to feeding difficulties in a number of ways that can coexist. Hypotonia can cause or exacerbate airway collapse by causing laxity in the muscular wall of the pharynx and the muscles of the larynx. The induction of any negative pressure into the upper or lower airway will be more likely to prompt collapse of the tissues if they have insufficient strength to maintain their normal position. Hypotonia will also make the mandible more likely to drop backward or open, both of which would reduce the anteroposterior diameter of the airway. Hypotonia may also affect feeding motions especially in neonates and infants, resulting in a weak suck or an inability to maintain sufficient oral suction for withdrawing milk from the breast or a bottle.

### Structural Anomalies of the Palate and Pharynx

Overt cleft palate affects the feeding process by making it impossible to create negative pressure in the oral cavity during feeding because the tongue cannot make an airtight seal with the palate (Sidoti & Shprintzen, 1995). In cases of submucous cleft palate and occult submucous cleft palate, the velopharyngeal valve, normally closed during swallowing, may not be able to seal completely, resulting in some nasal regurgitation of feedings. This is especially true in babies with VCFS because the pharynx is larger and deeper than normal, making it more difficult for a structurally abnormal palate to separate the nasopharynx from the oropharynx. Unfortunately, nasal regurgitation during feeding is often misinterpreted as reflux or simply labeled as reflux rather than regurgitation. Once the term reflux becomes attached to the baby, the typical reaction is often to prescribe antireflux medications such as proton pump inhibitors and antacids that may have been unnecessary. Asymmetry of the pharynx can cause compromise of the pyriform sinus on one side, preventing the bolus from flowing freely through it to the cricopharyngeus (Video 2–15), resulting in coughing or choking, and in the worst possible cases, aspiration. Another structural problem of the pharynx is prominent pulsation of the internal carotid artery that can make contact with the aryepiglottic fold, inducing a laryngeal adductor reflex, coughing, and choking (Video 2–16). These types of structural anomalies cannot be discerned without endoscopic examination of the upper airway or FEES (fiberoptic endoscopic evaluation of swallowing).

### Vascular Anomalies That Can Impinge on the Esophagus

Vascular anomalies can also affect the lower airway and esophagus. Abnormalities of the major vessels that branch from the aorta, such as the left and right subclavian arteries, or the aorta itself are common in VCFS. These aberrant vessels can take abnormal courses through the chest and impinge on the esophagus or the trachea. If the trachea is compressed, breathing is affected with a subsequent effect on feeding. If the esophagus is compressed, a stricture occurs so that a portion of a swallowed bolus can get hung up in the esophagus, prompting a reverse peristalsis and spitting up or emesis. As with nasal regurgitation, this esophageal rejection of a "not quite swallowed" bolus is often labeled as reflux and treated as such. The reality is that in this common malformation in VCFS, the food never reaches the stomach and is not reflux. Another common vascular malformation that can occur independent of congenital heart disease is vascular ring. Vascular ring is actually not a single malformation, but a grouping of abnormal vessels that encircle the esophagus and trachea. Sometimes the ring is comprised of a double aortic arch with one arch on each side of the trachea and esophagus that join again into a single vessel lower in the chest, with the result being a ring of vessels constricting the airway or esophagus. Another type of vascular ring is the association of a right-sided aortic arch (common in VCFS) with an aberrant right subclavian artery that combines to form a ring around the esophagus and trachea. The effect is the same regardless of the particular vessels involved. Vascular rings require surgical resolution. When not detected early, the strictures they cause can become permanent deformations of the trachea and esophagus.

### Slow Gastric Emptying

Although normative data are scarce, it has been generally accepted that an infant's stomach typically empties 40% of its contents after one hour and 60% after two hours (Heyman, Eicher, & Alavi, 1995). In hypotonic children and children who are constipated, emptying may be considerably delayed. As will be discussed later in this chapter, children with VCFS also grow at a different pace and follow a different growth curve than children who do not have VCFS. Therefore, when compared to normal growth curves, children with VCFS often fall below the norms for age. When this occurs, decisions are sometimes made to pursue hyperalimentation in order to increase growth. Increasing calories and volume of food intake will prompt discomfort from being overfilled and will likely increase spitting up and emesis and perhaps prompt gastroesophageal reflux. Rather than solving a growth problem (which hyperalimentation will not do), a new feeding problem is introduced because of discomfort associated with the feeding process. As will be discussed later (see Chapter 5), growth data and the diagnosis of failure-to-thrive need to be interpreted with a great deal of caution in children with VCFS to avoid making serious errors in judgment and treatment.

### Chronic Constipation

Clinicians who discuss feeding with parents must also obtain information about elimination and bowel movement patterns. A basic principle, crudely put, is that you cannot put food in one end if it does not come out of the other end. Most of us at one time or another have complained after a large meal that "if I eat one more bite, I'll explode." In some ways, this is not hyperbole. It is possible to eat too much and overfill the stomach, causing a physiologic explosion in the form of vomiting (the stomach's way of relieving abnormal internal pressure) and, if the problem persists for a long time, possible dumping syndrome. Because the gut clears slowly in VCFS, the infant may have persistent abdominal discomfort that will dull appetite. Resistance to feeding may be a sign of overfilling or abdominal discomfort, although many clinicians misinterpret avoidance, arching of the back, and irritability as a symptom of GER. This unfortunate judgment leads to treatment with medications before fully analyzing the entire feeding/elimination process from one end to the other (if you will pardon the humor). The preference is for babies to have at least one bowel movement per day (most newborns and infants have more). Relief of constipation often increases comfort and appetite, resulting not only in improved intake, but a happier baby.

### Irritable Temperament

It is difficult to feed well when you are unhappy. Temperament problems in VCFS are common (Antshel, Abdul Sabur, Roizen, Fremont, & Kates, 2006), and chronic illness and hospitalization can add to the problem. Children with VCFS are often labeled difficult and this behavior will generalize to feeding. Abdominal pain from constipation or overfilling will also lead to infantile irritability. Because babies with VCFS are often chronically ill and have persistent feeding problems and parents are concerned about the health and well-being, there may also be a tense and anxiety-provoking interaction between the baby and her parents. Feeding, instead of being a pleasant and warm process resulting in bonding between baby and parent, may become an anxiety-filled ritual where the goal is to get as much food into the baby so the baby will gain weight, rather than simply to make the baby content. This kind of anxiety-inducing situation during feeding could lead to even more irritability.

### Overall Constitutional Weakness Secondary to Congenital Heart Disease and Other Health Issues

Approximately 71% of newborns with VCFS have congenital heart disease, many with severe heart anomalies that can have a major effect on overall vitality and stamina. Babies with pulmonary stenosis or atresia in particular are at risk for feeding problems related to their strength and ability to stay awake during the feeding. Feedings tend to be shortened by the lack of vigor, therefore reducing oral intake.

### *Surgical Procedures*

Clinical experience has shown that many babies with VCFS have multiple surgical procedures associated with feeding. Early failure-to-thrive often results in the recommendation for gastrostomy. Gastrostomy tube feedings are often accompanied by hyperalimentation and constipation. Slow gastric emptying and hypotonia still exist, resulting in persistent spitting up that may still be interpreted as reflux. For some reason, nasal regurgitation is often interpreted as a risk for aspiration, although it is not. The persistent spitting up and nasal regurgitation may lead to the recommendation for Nissen fundal plication. Nissen fundal plications effectively prevent emesis and reflux, but this may not necessarily be a good thing in this situation. Spitting up and vomiting may be effective safety valves for preventing overfilling and abdominal discomfort. Once a Nissen is in place, the safety valve is no longer present. With a G-tube in place as well, the baby cannot refuse a feeding because no eating is involved. The feeding process is involuntary and is not associated with normal appetite and satiation, and the pleasure and happiness associated with eating meals with the family is not established. Once the G-tube is capped, there is no outlet except for the slow emptying that is common in VCFS, leaving the discomfort of a full stomach for an extended period of time. Retching and dry heaves are often experienced following G-tube feedings when a Nissen is in place. Prolonged hyperalimentation may then result in dumping syndrome. It should also be pointed out that gastrostomy tubes are often placed as a mechanism for getting babies out of the hospital more rapidly, rather than keeping the infant hospitalized for extended periods in order to establish feeding. Unfortunately, parents are often caught in the conundrum of hospitals not allowing discharge unless the baby is feeding but not allowing sufficient time to establish oral feeding because of the pressures of costly hospital stays.

## Failure-to-Thrive

Failure-to-thrive is a very nonspecific diagnostic term that is applied differently from one clinician to the next. One definition is as follows: "Failure to thrive is a description applied to children whose current weight or rate of weight gain is significantly below that of other children of similar age and sex" (Medline Plus, 2007). Another definition is: " . . . the failure to gain weight as expected, which is often accompanied by poor height growth" (Nemours Foundation, 2007). Still another is: "FTT is best defined as inadequate physical growth diagnosed by observation of growth over time using a standard growth chart" (American Academy of Family Physicians, 2007). These three definitions show the lack of standard definition for a term that often prompts serious treatments, including major surgery, in an attempt to improve feeding. The first definition focuses solely on weight as the indicator for failure-to-thrive. The second definition indicates poor weight gain as the focus, but goes further by saying that poor weight gain is accompanied by reduced height.

The third definition uses the term *growth* as the critical determining factor, but does not define growth, per se. Many children with VCFS have been seen who have been labeled as failure-to-thrive, although they were actually plump (Figure 2–66). Low weight for age is often the determining factor in diagnosing failure-to-thrive. However, low weight for age is based on normative data for the general population, such as the standardized CDC growth charts. Children with VCFS do not follow the "normal" growth velocities found in these charts, and weight distribution is different than in normal children. It is well known that genetic and chromosomal syndromes have their own growth curves, reflecting abnormal growth velocity. Children with Down syndrome do not follow the normal growth curves. Children with Turner syndrome do not follow the normal growth curves. Children with achondroplasia have their own growth curves that are normed for people with that particular genetic mutation. Why would one then think that children with a genetic disorder involving the deletion of 40 genes from chromosome 22 should be compared to the normal growth charts?

It is already known that children with VCFS are hypotonic and that the muscles have reduced mass (Shprintzen, 2005b; Zim et al., 2003). Muscle is a very dense and a heavier tissue than fat. Muscle is approximately 18% percent more dense than fat, and any reduction in muscle mass, even if replaced by fat, will mean a lower weight for height. Although it is not specifically known what percentage of muscle mass is lost in VCFS in relation to normal, it is clear that muscle mass is reduced in VCFS, so that body weight is proportionately lower, even if there is subcutaneous fat present. The presence of subcu-

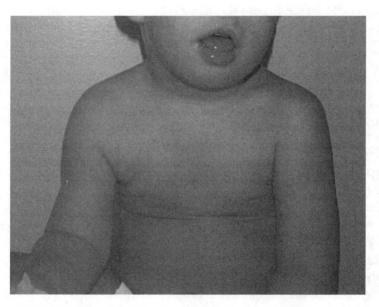

**FIGURE 2–66.** A child with VCFS who had been diagnosed with failure to thrive based on low weight for age.

taneous fat in humans means that more calories are being consumed than are required to support linear growth. Any calories not required to support linear growth or increase in muscle, skeletal, and brain development will be stored in the body as fat. Therefore, when children with VCFS are seen with deposits of subcutaneous fat, even if their weight has fallen off of the growth chart, the problem is not failure-to-thrive, but it is the chromosome deletion itself that causes a different rate of somatic growth than seen in the general population.

## Chronic Constipation

Constipation is a common and persistent problem in children with VCFS. In some cases, constipation can be caused by anal anomalies that prevent easy elimination. Imperforate anus and abnormal location of the anus (usually anterior displacement) can occur in VCFS and these anomalies may restrict bowel movements secondary to abnormal anatomy. However, in most cases, constipation in children with VCFS is related to overall muscle tone issues, and this type of problem is not uncommon in children with hypotonicity who have other multiple anomaly syndromes. A bowel that fails to empty at a normal rate will cause abdominal discomfort and reduce appetite. It will also result in slow gastric emptying. If the stomach empties slowly, the child will not want to eat and will also be more likely to spit up or vomit. It is therefore important to treat constipation effectively in children with VCFS in order to improve their desire to eat. The presence of chronic constipation often leads clinicians to suspect Hirschsprung aganglionic megacolon (sometimes known as Hirschsprung disease). Hirschsprung aganglionic megacolon is a condition in which ganglion cells that supply innervation to the colon are deficient, resulting in reduced peristaltic activity. The more time it takes for the stool to move through the bowel, the more water is extracted from it, making it harder and thereby increasing the risk of impaction. A single case of Hirschsprung aganglionic megacolon has been reported in association with VCFS (Kerstjens-Frederikse, Hofstra, van Essen, Meijers, & Buys, 1999), and it is unclear at this time if this case represents a chance occurrence or a syndromic association. However, if the Hirschsprung is a syndromic feature, then it would seem to be an uncommon one.

## Gastroesophageal Reflux

Gastroesophageal reflux is also known by the acronym GER, and when chronic and persistent (two or more episodes per week), the acronym GERD (gastroesophageal reflux disease) is applied. Diagnosing GER or GERD is a bit problematic because the symptoms are nonspecific and occur in many clinical conditions. Most people regard a pH probe as the gold standard diagnostic procedure for GERD, but the procedure is invasive and uncomfortable for young children. Therefore, many clinicians choose to treat GERD empirically by using antireflux medications, antacids, or proton pump inhibitors (PPIs). If one medication fails, multiple medications are often applied. Therefore, the true prevalence of GER or GERD in VCFS is not known at this time. In addition, because esophageal strictures and compressions are common in VCFS, it is not clear if GER is a label legitimately attached when the material irritating the esophagus is stomach contents or food that has never made it to the stomach.

Spitting up or nasal regurgitation is often misdiagnosed as GER or GERD. This semantic error is not trivial because it may lead to incorrect treatments being applied. Although GER can be extraesophageal (i.e., leaves the esophagus), the large majority of instances of GER are limited to the esophagus itself.

## Nasal Regurgitation

Nasal regurgitation is a common finding in VCFS in the neonatal period, often lasting through infancy and early childhood. Nasal regurgitation has several physiologic and anatomic causes in VCFS. Many clinicians erroneously regard nasal regurgitation as a dangerous clinical finding with specific concerns that this problem may lead to aspiration. Part of the problem is that the term *nasal reflux* is often assigned to this finding, but it is not reflux. It may be emesis or a bolus that has become entrapped in the esophagus because of a stricture or compression. Emesis may also occur following overfilling of the stomach. The only difference between nasal regurgitation and spitting up through the mouth is the route of the vomitus. Nasal regurgitation occurs in VCFS for a number of reasons related to velopharyngeal insufficiency, including palatal anomalies, platybasia leading to increased pharyngeal depth, and hypotonia. Although common and possibly alarming to parents, nasal regurgitation is not a source of concern in terms of increased risk of aspiration or airway compromise. If the normal protective mechanisms are in place, meaning a normal laryngeal adductor reflex that prevents aspiration, nasal regurgitation should not cause major concern.

Palatal anomalies in VCFS occur in approximately 75% of cases ranging from overt palatal clefts to occult submucous cleft and asymmetric palate. Nasal regurgitation should not be a surprise in these cases, because this problem is seen in otherwise normal children who have the same palatal anomalies. This is especially true for infants with overt palatal clefts, although it is common in submucous clefts as well. When hypotonicity of the velopharyngeal musculature is added to the process, as is true in VCFS, nasal regurgitation is essentially inevitable.

Platybasia plays a role because the size of the nasopharynx is increased in VCFS (Golding-Kushner, 1991; Zim et al., 2003). Therefore, when spitting up or emesis occurs, the vomitus may follow the path of least resistance towards the largest part of the pharynx. This is simple fluid dynamics, and because nasopharyngeal size is increased in VCFS, there should be no sur-prise that the nasopharynx would fill more easily than in normal infants, resulting in nasal regurgitation.

## Irritability

Irritability in infants is often interpreted as being secondary to other problems that would be considered to be unpleasant. It is a natural inclina-tion to correlate two findings, such as a feeding problem with irritability, and to think that there is a cause and effect relationship. Although correlations can imply cause and effect interactions, the direction of that interaction is not always obvious. It is also true that there are many things that have perfect cor-relations that do not have cause and effect relationships, for example, Mon-day and Tuesday. Monday does not cause Tuesday, and Tuesday does not cause Monday, but they do occur in the same order 100% of the time, a perfect 1.0 correlation. The relationship between Monday and Tuesday is caused by a third influence, the calendar. Whoever devised the calendar and arranged the days by name caused the relationship to be a perfect correlation. Therefore, in relation to VCFS and infantile irritability, there are several possibilities. One is that feeding problems cause irritability. The second is that irritability causes the child to be unhappy during feedings and therefore less likely to feed. And, of course, both of these things may be true (a bidirectional correlation). The third possibility is that there is no cause and effect relationship but that both the irritability and feeding problems are caused by the deletion from chromo-some 22. Temperament is a biologically determined component of behavior and is evident even in infancy. Temperament abnormalities have been docu-mented in VCFS, and it is likely that they are interpreted as irritability and babies being "difficult," which is also the case in childhood (Antshel et al., 2007). It is important to recognize temperament issues in VCFS to prevent incorrect assumptions about the cause of irritability that might lead to unnec-essary medical management of those presumed problems.

## GENITOURINARY ANOMALIES

Anomalies of the genitals and the urinary tract are common in VCFS, but they are not typically of major impact on quality of life. They include:

125. Hypospadias

126. Cryptorchidism

127. Vesicoureteral reflux

128. Hydrocele

## Hypospadias

Hypospadias is an anomaly of the penis and therefore occurs only in males. Its frequency in VCFS is approximately 14% of affected males (Shprintzen, 1999). Hypospadias is a fusion anomaly of the penis in which the urethral opening is not at the tip of the penis but on the underside (Figure 2–67). Hypospadias is usually treated with elective surgery for functional and esthetic reasons, but it does not typically affect urination except for an abnormal path for the stream.

## Cryptorchidism

Cryptorchidism, or undescended testicles, is the most common genital anomaly in humans. Although approximately 3% of newborns have one or both testes undescended at birth, the number is reduced to 1% by 1 year of age because most cases resolve spontaneously (Pettersson, Richiardi, Nordenskjold, Kaijser, & Akre, 2007). It occurs in approximately 18% of males with VCFS (Shprintzen, 1999). Cryptorchidism often occurs in the same individuals who have hypospadias and is also more common among people with inguinal hernias. When left untreated, there is an increased risk of testicular cancer. Orchiopexy, a surgical procedure, is recommended before puberty (Pettersson et al., 2007).

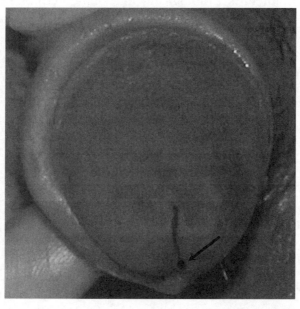

**FIGURE 2–67.** Hypospadias in a male with VCFS.

## Vesicoureteral Reflux

Vesicoureteral reflux (VUR) is relatively common in VCFS. In VUR, some urine backs up through the ureters so that, instead of draining into the bladder for elimination, it may return to the kidneys. The danger of VUR is the instigation of urinary tract infections (UTI) or renal infections that might cause permanent kidney damage, or renal failure that can result in hypertension. Because of the risk of UTI and the overall problems of immune disorder or deficiency in VCFS, some patients may be treated with antibiotic prophylaxis. In most cases, VUR improves and resolves over time. In rare cases, surgery may be necessary to prevent VUR.

## Hydrocele

A hydrocele is a fluid-filled sac in the scrotum that runs along the spermatic cord. Hydroceles are common isolated anomalies in the general population, but more common in VCFS. Hydroceles often occur together with inguinal hernias. When isolated anomalies, most hydroceles resolve spontaneously and do not require surgical management. When they persist, or when they are associated with inguinal hernias, they do require surgical correction.

# SKELETAL, MUSCLE, SPINAL, AND ORTHOPEDIC ANOMALIES

VCFS has a large number of anomalies of the skeleton, skeletal muscles, and spine that may require orthopedic intervention. In many cases, however, treatment is not indicated and the problems presented are chronic but not debilitating. These problems include:

129. Scoliosis

130. Vertebral anomalies

131. Spina bifida occulta

132. Syrinx

133. Tethered cord

134. Osteopenia

135. Sprengel anomaly

136. Talipes equinovarus and valgus deformity

137. Hypoplastic skeletal muscles

138. Hyperextensible/lax joints

139. Joint dislocations

140. Flat foot arches

141. Chronic leg pains

142. Extra ribs, rib fusion

## Scoliosis

Scoliosis is an abnormal curvature of the spine. Scoliosis occurs in approximately 30% of individuals with VCFS. In scoliosis, the spine curves to one side or the other. In VCFS, the curvature is almost always to the right and is typically in the thoracic spine. For people with scoliosis who do not have VCFS, the curvatures are also typically to the right. The frequency of scoliosis in VCFS is approximately 15 times greater than seen in the general population. The specific reason for the development of scoliosis in VCFS is unknown. It is not clear if spine anomalies, hypotonia, or a primary genetic influence play a role. The problem may be present in childhood, but most often becomes apparent at or just after the onset of puberty simultaneous to the pubertal growth spurt. Treatment options are limited. In nonsyndromic individuals, scoliosis is tracked clinically and by spine radiographs. When the curvature becomes severe enough or symptomatic in terms of pain, bracing is begun. If bracing fails to resolve the problem or at least hold it in check, surgery (spinal fusion) is recommended. Clinical experience has shown that bracing is not effective in VCFS. Those cases with progressive curvature tend to worsen rapidly after the onset of puberty. Because people with VCFS have both pulmonary and cardiac problems, careful follow-up of scoliosis is warranted and surgery is indicated in those cases of clinical significance.

## Vertebral Anomalies

Vertebral malformations have been reported in VCFS (Ricchetti et al., 2004), including fusion of cervical spine vertebrae, anomalies of the atlas, and abnormal motion of the vertebrae. Clinical observations also include butterfly vertebrae, hemivertebrae, and spina bifida occulta (see below). Limitation of head turn, low posterior hairline, and short neck may be clues to spinal anomalies and would be clear indication for spine radiographs. The question remains as to the imperative for routine spinal studies for all individuals with VCFS. However, because there is a relatively high frequency of scoliosis in VCFS, baseline spine radiographs are probably a good idea for all children with VCFS.

## Spina Bifida Occulta

Spina bifida refers to a malformation of the spine where there is incomplete development or a small gap in one or more of the vertebrae. Although any of the vertebrae may be anomalous, the most commonly affected bones are in the lower spine. A diagnostic clue may be the presence of a pilonidal dimple or pit (Figure 2–68). Most children with spina bifida occulta have no functional abnormalities or neurological problems. In rare cases, there is a complete spina bifida of the vertebrae, which will be discussed later in relation to several rare cases of meningomyelocele that have been reported in VCFS. Although not a clinical problem, the presence of spinal column anomalies may imply some primary developmental disorders associated with the neural tube, therefore pointing towards some contribution from the deletion at 22q11.2.

## Syrinx

A syrinx is a fluid-filled space in the spinal cord. A syrinx may be a congenital anomaly, as it is in VCFS, or caused by trauma. Although not a common anomaly in VCFS, syrinx has been seen frequently enough in our population to

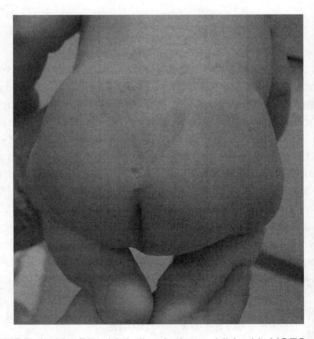

**FIGURE 2–68.** Pilonidal dimple in a child with VCFS who has spina bifida occulta and a tethered cord.

identify it as a feature of VCFS. It is possible that our detection of syrinx in VCFS is related to the fact that most of our patients at The VCFS International Center at Upstate Medical University have MRI studies of the spine. In most cases, the syrinx is not symptomatic, but syrinx can expand with time, resulting in damage to the center of the spinal cord. If the nerve fibers in the spinal cord are damaged, symptoms may develop according to the severity and location of the syrinx. Limb weakness, loss of bowel and bladder control, and loss of temperature sensation are among the sensory and motor problems that can occur if a syrinx results in significant spinal cord damage. Therefore, detection with careful follow-up is indicated.

### Tethered Cord

Tethered cord refers to an abnormal attachment of the spinal cord to one or more vertebrae. Tethered cord has been seen in a small number of cases of children with VCFS, but at a rate far higher than expected in the general population. This anomaly occurs at the base of the spine in VCFS and may be asymptomatic. Tethered cord often occurs in association with spina bifida occulta. Possible symptoms caused by tethered cord include loss of bowel and bladder control, back pain, loss of sensation in the feet and/or legs, and weakness in the legs. The presence of a pilonidal dimple (Figure 2–68) may also be a diagnostic clue to the presence of a tethered cord.

### Osteopenia

Osteopenia is a decrease in bone mineral density that is below normal, but not so abnormally low as to be classified as osteoporosis. However, people with osteopenia are at risk for the development of osteoporosis. In other words, osteopenia is not characterized by bone loss, whereas osteoporosis is. Osteopenia is asymptomatic but can be detected with bone scans. Because osteopenia can be treated with calcium and vitamin D supplements, detecting it early is of importance. In VCFS, osteopenia typically becomes evident in adolescence and is more common in females, but males may also be affected. Although not a common finding in VCFS, it is clearly underdetected because bone scans are not a normal part of child or adolescent health assessments. Bone scans are recommended in adolescents with VCFS, especially if there has been a positive history in the past of hypocalcemia, but absence of documented hypocalcemia does not rule out the possible development of osteopenia.

### Sprengel Anomaly

Sprengel anomaly, also known as Sprengel shoulder, refers to a vertical displacement of the scapula high on the back above the normal placement

(Figure 2–69). Sprengel anomaly has no functional significance and treatment is not required, although some people have requested surgical correction for cosmetic reasons. However, the presence of Sprengel anomaly may have diagnostic significance for VCFS in individuals without other characteristic signs of the syndrome.

### Talipes Equinovarus and Valgus Deformity

Talipes equinovarus is also known as club foot and involves the torsion of the foot inwards. Talipes equinovarus may be caused by intrauterine constraint, as in a breech position during pregnancy, and in such cases, casting and external physical forces will correct the problem. In the case of VCFS, the anomaly is likely caused by either vascular anomalies or neurogenic ones related to the neural tube. A link between neural tube defects and club foot is well known, and given the occurrence of tethered cord, syrinx, and other neural tube anomalies in VCFS, this may be responsible for some or all cases of talipes equinovarus. Club foot can also be caused by restricted perfusion to the foot

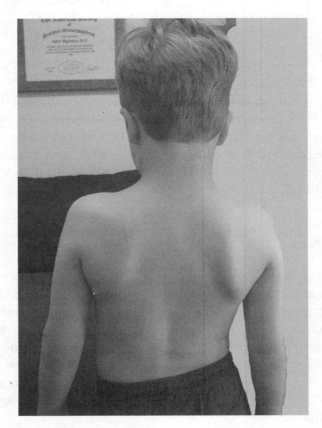

**FIGURE 2–69.** Sprengel shoulder in a child with VCFS.

that fails to drive growth of the affected side. Vascular problems are also common in VCFS. A vascular explanation makes sense in VCFS because valgus deformities of the foot (torsion of the foot in the opposite direction of a club foot) also occur. The precise cause of club foot is unknown in VCFS. Fortunately, this is a relatively low frequency anomaly in VCFS. Surgical correction of club foot or a valgus deformity is often necessary when not caused by external physical constraint.

## Hypoplastic Skeletal Muscles

Hypoplasia of the muscle tissue in the pharynx and palate in VCFS has been demonstrated histologically (Zim et al., 2003). Similar data do not exist for other muscle groups, but hypotonia of the limbs, face, and trunk is well known in VCFS, and children with VCFS do not appear to be as well muscled as their peers. Besides the relationship of muscle mass to weight as previously discussed, hypoplastic skeletal muscles will affect overall physical strength and coordination, motor development, and levels of physical activity. It is likely that the deletion of one or more of the genes from 22q11.2 results in decreased muscle mass, and several of the genes are known to be highly expressed in skeletal muscle.

## Hyperextensible/Lax Joints

The large and small joints (elbows, knees, hips, fingers, toes, etc.) are hyperextensible in the majority of children with VCFS. Checking for joint laxity is one of the methods for diagnosing hypotonia. Although some children have joint laxity because of connective tissue dysplasia, as in Marfan syndrome, Stickler syndrome, and Ehlers-Danlos syndrome, the problem in VCFS is related to abnormal muscle tone.

## Joint Dislocations

Joint dislocations are not common in people with VCFS, but they do occur on occasion and are secondary to joint laxity and low muscle tone. When the joints are hyperextensible and the muscles do not provide sufficient resistance against external forces, then the joints are more likely to yield to those forces, making it easier for them to dislocate. Clinical experience has yielded cases with dislocated elbows and knees, but only on a few occasions in patients who were more severely hypotonic. This is not a common occurrence and should not prevent children with VCFS from participating in physical exercise or athletics.

## Flat Foot Arches

Although flat feet is a common finding in the general population, it is nearly ubiquitous in VCFS. In fact, the only cases encountered who did not have flat foot arches had abnormally high arches, but these cases were few in number and represent a different problem with a similar cause. Low muscle tone typically makes the foot pronate when standing. The foot arch cannot be assessed with the patient is sitting on an examination table or in a chair. The foot arches typically look normal when the foot is in a relaxed state and not bearing the body's weight. When children with VCFS stand, the arch flattens and the foot turns out, known as pronation, causing abnormal stretch of the muscles in the lower leg (Figure 2–70). In some cases, the foot compensates in the other direction, with the foot arch becoming higher so that the child bears weight on the outside of the foot. This also causes abnormal stretching

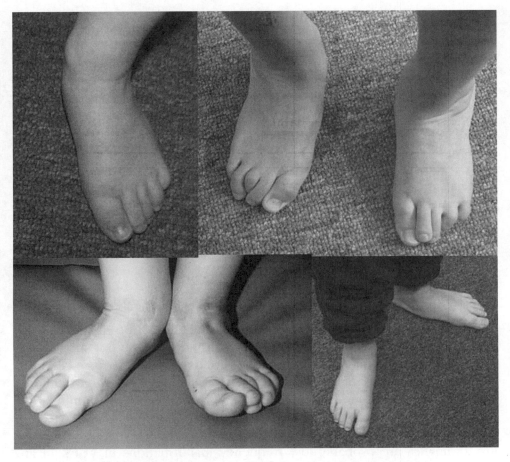

**FIGURE 2–70.** Flat feet in VCFS showing marked pronation.

of the same muscles, although with a different torsion. The effect, however, is the same.

Flat foot arches are a potential source of chronic pain and therefore require attention. Because flat foot arches are a very common problem in VCFS, parents should be aware of the need for appropriate footwear for their children, and in some cases, the need for arch support. Arch support should be soft enough to yield to the pressure of the foot while still keeping the arch in a normal position. Rigid inserts tend to cause discomfort because the child will often posture the foot abnormally in order to avoid walking on a hard surface that is curved up towards the instep. A more gentle support is preferred. Good running shoes with a palpable rubbery rise at the instep are the best shoes for children with VCFS because they are comfortable to wear and provide good arch support. If additional arch support is needed, latex rubber inserts molded to the foot are best. Supports known as cobra pads have been recommended for this purpose (Al-Khattat, 2007).

## Chronic Leg Pains

Research has shown that a high percentage of children with VCFS, approximately half, experience chronic leg pains (Shprintzen, 1999; Al-Khattat, 2007). Although some children verbalize discomfort, younger children may not be able to do so but may give signals that indicate the problem. These include asking to be picked up while walking, sleep disturbance, kicking during sleep, irritability, and refusal to engage in exercise. At night, when the child is in bed and off of the feet, cramps will occur as the muscles that have been stretched in abnormal positions all day return to their normal position. The resulting contractions of those muscles may cause discomfort or even sharp pain that disturbs sleep or prevents the child from falling asleep. A program of stretching, massage, and wearing proper footwear will resolve these pains.

## Extra Ribs, Rib Fusions

Rib anomalies have been reported in approximately 17% of individuals with VCFS (Ming et al., 1997), although our own clinical data do not support this frequency. It is possible that rib anomalies are undetected because clinicians are not typically looking for them. However, a large percentage of children with VCFS do have chest or torso radiographs because of pneumonia and other lower respiratory illnesses, congenital heart disease, and scoliosis. It is likely that in some or most cases anomalies of the rib cage would be detected. Rib anomalies are probably low frequency malformations in VCFS. In any event, they are not functionally significant.

## SKIN AND HAIR FINDINGS

In addition to the rough skin and morphea found specifically on the hands and feet, there are two additional minor findings:

143. Abundant scalp hair

144. Thin appearing skin (venous patterns easily visible)

### Abundant Scalp Hair

As was noted in the original article published about VCFS in 1978 (Shprintzen et al., 1978), the scalp tends to have abundant hair. Occasionally, the scalp hair looks dense because there are a normal number of hair follicles on the head of someone with microcephaly (a small head). The scalp would therefore have less surface area and the normal number of follicles would make the hair look denser. An analysis of the number of hair follicles per square centimeter has not been done for VCFS, so at this point, the abundant scalp hair is simply an interesting observation that may assist in the diagnosis of the syndrome.

### Thin Appearing Skin

The skin over the arms, legs, torso, and back seems to be thin in people with VCFS. It is unclear if the appearance of the skin means that the skin is of normal thickness but more translucent, or if the layers of skin are actually thinner. When examining the skin in VCFS, venous patterns are easily visible, and any degree of venous congestion becomes readily apparent. There is no known significance of this finding at this time.

## ENDOCRINE AND IMMUNE FINDINGS

When initially reported by Angelo DiGeorge in 1968, the major emphasis on the DiGeorge sequence was on the endocrine findings. This is certainly understandable given that DiGeorge is a pediatric endocrinologist. Although there are a number of endocrine findings associated with VCFS, the one that was first identified by DiGeorge and that draws the most attention is hypoparathyroidism. However, there are other endocrine findings that are more common and more important in the long-term management of VCFS than hypoparathyroidism. The endocrine anomalies associated with VCFS include:

145. Hypocalcemia

146. Hypoparathyroidism

147. Hypothyroidism/hyperthyroidism/autoimmune thyroiditis

148. Hypoglycemia

149. Mild growth deficiency, relatively small stature (childhood)

150. Absent, hypoplastic thymus

151. Small pituitary gland (rare)

152. Immune deficiency or immune disorder

## Hypocalcemia

People need calcium for a number of important functions in the body. Although many minerals (such as calcium, sodium, potassium, and magnesium) are necessary for maintaining good health, calcium deserves special attention because it is the most plentiful mineral found in the human body. Calcium is primarily associated with our bones and teeth because the basic substance of bone and enamel are calcium rich. However, calcium is also needed for muscle function and the proper functioning of the kidneys and lymphatic system. The body maintains a relatively constant balance of essential minerals for normal cellular function. In order for cell membranes and other tissues to function properly for the exchange of ions that are essential to the workings of the body, the body has to have these mineral ions available. Hypocalcemia, either transient or persistent, is present in approximately one quarter of individuals with VCFS (Shprintzen, 1999). This may be an underestimate for a number of reasons. First, in most cases of VCFS, hypocalcemia is transient. When serum calcium levels are measured, they may be normal at times, but abnormal at other times. Calcium levels fall when a person is under stress or when dehydrated or engaging in physical exercise. Calcium is typically measured during a routinely scheduled doctor's appointment when these factors are not in operation. It is also true that hypocalcemia varies with age in VCFS. Low calcium levels are often detected in infancy, especially after open-heart surgery, and then normalize, and then they may return in teen years after the onset of puberty. It is therefore recommended that serum calcium and ionized calcium levels be measured at least annually throughout life in people with VCFS. It is also important that people with VCFS get enough sunlight and have sufficient vitamin D in their diets. Calcium cannot be utilized properly without vitamin D, and vitamin D requires sunlight to be activated. Normal calcium levels are also maintained by parathyroid hormone.

In its most severe forms, hypocalcemia can result in hypocalcemic seizures (because of the importance of calcium to brain cell function). When calcium levels drop, the neurons that activate muscles become more excitable, resulting in hypocalcemic seizures. Symptoms include numbness and tingling of the extremities and the area around the mouth, muscle cramping and muscle stiffness, spasms of the arms and legs, and tremors.

Although often seen in infancy, cases have been seen that presented initially in the late teens or early adult years. In such cases, hypocalcemia or hypoparathyroidism had not been documented previously. The mechanism for this late onset of hypocalcemia is not understood as yet. Plotting calcium levels throughout life for individuals with VCFS will be important in terms of understanding why cases of hypocalcemia present at specific ages.

## Hypoparathyroidism

The parathyroid glands are four glands, two under each lateral portion of the thyroid gland arranged top and bottom. These glands secrete parathyroid hormone (PTH), which is essential in the body's proper use of calcium and phosphorous. The presence of hypocalcemia, even when transient, should suggest that PTH be assessed. Hypoparathyroidism is not actually very common in VCFS, probably occurring in less than 10% of the total number of cases. However, it was hypoparathyroidism that led Angelo DiGeorge to describe the condition in association with congenital heart disease and immune deficiency (DiGeorge, 1968). The only symptom of hypoparathyroidism is hypocalcemia. The other findings described by DiGeorge are part of a developmental sequence (see Chapter 1, Box 1). The relationship between the parathyroid glands, immune deficiency, and congenital heart disease has to relate back to a single embryonic error of development that has a cascading effect on subsequent embryonic development.

## Hypothyroidism/Hyperthyroidism/Autoimmune Thyroiditis

More common than hypoparathyroidism is hypothyroidism and other thyroid disorders. The most common thyroid problem is hypothyroidism, which typically appears in early adolescence, typically close to the onset of puberty. However, hypothyroidism has been seen in young children, as early as 4 or 5 years of age. Screening for thyroid disease is recommended at each well child examination that the child has on an annual basis. Hypothyroidism can be a serious and confusing problem in VCFS because of an overlap of symptoms with some of the other phenotypes associated with VCFS. These include fatigue, constipation, depression, joint and muscle pain, dry skin, and hoarseness. Because the manifestations of hypothyroidism can masquerade as psychiatric illness, it becomes important to check for thyroid disease on a regular basis to be certain that treatment is focused on the right system.

In some cases, patients with VCFS develop Graves' disease or Hashimoto's thyroiditis, both of them forms of autoimmune response (Choi et al., 2005; Gosselin, Lebon-Labich, Lucron, Marçon, & Leheup, 2004; Kawame et al., 2001). Graves' disease is the opposite of hypothyroidism in that the thyroid become overactive. The symptoms are similar in part to hypothyroidism in that there is chronic fatigue and irritability. However, instead of constipation, there is an increase in frequency of bowel movements, and rather than weight gain there is weight loss. Hashimoto's thyroiditis results in hypothyroidism. Both Graves' and Hashimoto's are the result of chronic inflammation of the thyroid gland that is an autoimmune response, meaning that the body's immune system attacks its own tissues and organs as if they were invading germs or viruses, thereby irritating or destroying the tissue. It is possible that most or all thyroid disorders in VCFS represent an autoimmune response. Hashimoto's thyroiditis has been linked to hypoparathyroidism, but it is not known if this is the case in individuals with VCFS.

## Hypoglycemia

Although not reported in the literature, hypoglycemia can occur in VCFS, and several cases have been seen in our program, including infants and young children. The cause in these cases is not known, but hypoglycemia can be caused by other imbalances in the endocrine system. Hypoglycemia can also be a response to stress, chronic illness, surgery, renal anomalies, and even severe anxiety. Hypoglycemia can sometimes be a challenge with children with VCFS because eating may be problematic. Eating disorders are common in VCFS, especially with early mismanagement, unnecessary surgery, and discomfort induced by attempted hyperalimentation. The potential risk of hypoglycemia might result in the recommendation for alternative feeding methods, such as the placement of a G-tube, but the preference should always be for normal eating and, if hypoglycemia is detected, recommending frequent small meals during the day to keep blood sugar at normal levels.

## Mild Growth Deficiency, Relatively Small Stature in Childhood

In initial reports describing VCFS, short stature was described as a clinical feature (Goldberg, Motzkin, Marion, Scambler, & Shprintzen, 1993; Motzkin, Marion, Goldberg, Shprintzen, & Saenger, 1993; Ryan et al., 1997; Shprintzen, Goldberg, Young, & Wolford, 1981). The frequency of short stature in these reports ranged from 29 to 50%. All of these studies relied on cross-sectional data obtained almost exclusively from young children. As more adults with VCFS were diagnosed and as more longitudinal experience was developed so that young patients initially diagnosed were seen in adult years, it became evident that VCFS is not a syndrome that results in short stature in adult life in most cases. Because we began studying VCFS in 1975 prior to the first publication about the syndrome (Shprintzen et al., 1978), many of the cases we saw at that time are now adults in their 40s, 50s, and several older. It became apparent after seeing more than 50 adults with VCFS that they were not abnormally short. Two questions remained. Were they short in relation to "expected height" (sometimes referred to as mid-parental height, which is the measure often used to predict a child's height on reaching adulthood), and if short stature occurred in younger children with VCFS, did that continue into adult life, so that these children remained short? The problem with cross-sectional growth data is that children with VCFS are compared to growth curves that are based on the general population for chronological age. It is possible that people with VCFS have a different growth velocity that does not compare well to the growth velocity of people who do not have VCFS. For example, there are separate growth curves for Down syndrome, achondroplasia, and other genetic conditions that have short stature as a consistent feature, but it is not simply that the terminus of their growth curve is below the norm. The velocity and rate of growth are also different for these syndromes as well as many others. If children with VCFS have different growth velocities than normal, then it is possible that they would be classified as short of stature at 5 years of age, but not at 18. It was therefore necessary to develop a growth curve specific to VCFS that included longitudinal data. A preliminary growth curve for VCFS is shown in Chapter 5. The results of our study show that the majority of people with VCFS reach mid-parental height, although females tend to be a bit shorter as a group compared to males. Although children with VCFS are often smaller than their peers through childhood because of the difference in their growth velocity, they tend to catch up by the time they reach late adolescence. Very few patients with VCFS have been treated with growth hormone in order to resolve short stature, the percentage being no different than that seen in the general population.

## Absent, Hypoplastic Thymus

The thymus gland is a bilobed gland that sits in the center of the chest in close proximity to the heart, often covering it. The thymus plays a role in immunologic response and by producing T-lymphocytes, white blood cells that respond to fight infections. The *T* in T-lymphocytes implies that the cell is thymus derived. Although the thymus is typically located over the heart, there is often thymic tissue elsewhere in the chest or sometimes in the neck. Because babies with VCFS often require open-heart surgery and the thymus covers the heart, surgeons often have to remove the thymus in order to access the heart. It is interesting to note that these patients do not typically have severe immune deficiency. It is therefore likely that thymic tissue is present elsewhere in the body or that there are other mechanisms for producing T cells outside of the thymus. The embryologic history of the thymus is one of migrating from the neck to the chest, and in many cases, thymic tissue continues to line this path after birth. Ultrasound study has found that more than 60% of children have thymic tissue in the neck (Chu & Metreweli, 2002).

## Small Pituitary Gland

Pituitary hypoplasia or aplasia can occur in VCFS, but it is a rare anomaly. Midline brain anomalies such as holoprosencephaly (Wraith et al., 1985), signaling severe morphologic errors in formation, have been noted in VCFS, and in such cases the pituitary gland is always absent. Absence of the pituitary has implications for growth because of the absence of pituitary growth hormone. In cases where the pituitary is absent, the brain should be checked for anomalies, and the sense of smell should be checked for anosmia.

## Immune Deficiency or Immune Disorder

Because immune deficiency was part of the phenotype initially described by DiGeorge and others, immunologic problems are considered to be a major feature of VCFS. True immune deficiency is actually relatively rare in VCFS. Immune deficiency is a life-threatening disorder defined by laboratory analyses that show significantly reduced populations of the cells that fight invading microbes and, more importantly, clear evidence that the cells that are present do not function normally. People with immune deficiency have reduced populations of T-lymphocytes, specifically low numbers of CD4 and CD8 cells. CD4 cells, also known as helper cells, $T_h$, or effector cells, do not directly attack bacteria or viruses, but they act to activate and direct other lymphocytes to kill microbes. CD8 cells, also known as $CD8^+T$ cells, attach to cells that have been infected with viruses and kill those cells before the viruses in it can reproduce and be released to infect more cells.

Some children with VCFS have reduced populations of lymphocytes on laboratory analysis, but the cells that are present function normally. In such cases, there may be little or no effect on the immune system. In many cases, however, there are more frequent upper respiratory infections, and those that occur may last longer, but eventually with age the immune system tends to respond normally as antibodies are formed to common illnesses. It is also possible to have normal populations of T cells but the cells do not function normally. This is a less common but more dangerous situation in that it results in a true immune deficiency.

The presence of lower respiratory infections in infancy or early childhood is a strong warning signal that an immune disorder is present. Children with VCFS who develop pneumonia or bronchitis early in life are likely to have them again later in life. In such cases, early childhood may be a period of multiple respiratory illnesses ranging from middle ear disease to pneumonia. Pneumonias can be particularly difficult to interpret and manage in VCFS because some clinicians consider feeding difficulties and nasal regurgitation as a risk for aspiration. In addition, many children with VCFS have chronic respiratory irritation, often diagnosed as reactive airway disease or asthma.

The majority of children with VCFS have more respiratory illnesses than their peers, but few have the debilitating immune deficiency that can be life threatening. In fact, more children with VCFS have normal immune responses than have severe immune deficiency. In those children with frequent respiratory illnesses, the typical picture is for them to decrease in both severity and frequency over time, most typically after 6 or 7 years of age.

## SPEECH AND LANGUAGE DISORDERS

Among the most common of problems in VCFS is communication impairment. The recognition of the syndrome has been largely based on the presence of severe hypernasality (Sedláčková, 1955; Shprintzen et al., 1978). The speech disorders, language impairment, and the reason for velopharyngeal insufficiency have been extensively studied and reported (Arvystas & Shprintzen, 1984; Chegar et al., 2006; Chegar, Shprintzen, Curtis, & Tatum, 2007; Golding-Kushner, 1991; Golding-Kushner et al., 1985; Havkin et al., 2000; Shprintzen, 1982; Shprintzen, 2000a; Shprintzen et al., 1978; Shprintzen, Goldberg, Golding-Kushner, & Marion, 1992; Tatum et al., 2002; Williams et al., 1987; Zim et al., 2003). Because these issues have been so well defined, the results have been immediately applied to treatment outcomes, an example of true translational research. Communicative disorders include:

153. Velopharyngeal insufficiency (usually severe)

154. Severe hypernasality

155. Severe articulation impairment (glottal stops)

156. High pitched voice

157. Hoarseness

158. Language impairment (usually mild delay)

### Velopharyngeal Insufficiency (VPI)

As described earlier in this chapter, the functioning of the velopharyngeal mechanism can be disordered by multiple factors that include structural palate anomalies, an excessively deep pharynx with a large volume, pharyngeal hypotonia, pharyngeal asymmetry, abnormal pharyngeal musculature, and a hypoplastic or aplastic adenoid. Some or all of these anomalies could be present in a single individual. Although many clinicians focus on the palatal anomalies (overt, submucous, or occult submucous cleft) as being the primary cause of VPI, this is not the case. It must be pointed out that the majority of people who do not have VCFS but who have repaired clefts of the palate or unrepaired submucous clefts have normal speech (Gereau & Shprintzen, 1988; Salyer, Song, & Sperry, 2006; Shprintzen et al., 1985). However, children with VCFS who have repaired clefts or unrepaired submucous clefts with rare exception have severely hypernasal speech. There is clearly something different about VPI in VCFS than in other populations with palatal anomalies.

When the palate is considered separate from its surroundings, it is not possible to fully understand why the velopharyngeal valve dysfunctions. Studies have shown that the volume of the pharynx in individuals with VCFS is much larger than normal (Shprintzen, 1982; Golding-Kushner, 1991) and that the volume is often increased because the adenoid is small or absent (Williams et al., 1987). The lateral pharyngeal walls are also more laterally displaced (Shprintzen, 1982) and move poorly, if at all (Golding-Kushner, 1991). Therefore, in order for the palate to occlude the pharynx, the movement of the palate needs to be greater than it might be if it were contained within a pharynx of normal dimension. The lateral pharyngeal walls would also have to move towards the pharyngeal midline sufficiently to occlude the lateral aspects of the pharynx, which are also larger than normal.

Although the demand for increased movement is present, the capacity for it in VCFS is also diminished. Hypotonia of the pharynx and palate is very common in VCFS, caused by abnormal musculature (Zim et al., 2003). The pharyngeal muscles in VCFS are hypoplastic and have an abnormal distribution of type 1 and type 2 fibers, and the muscle fibers themselves are abnormally small (Zim et al., 2003). The thickness of the pharyngeal walls and palate is also known to be abnormally small (Golding-Kushner, 1991; Zim et al., 2003).

The posterior pharyngeal wall is also positioned abnormally in relation to the palate secondary to platybasia, which has the effect of moving the posterior pharyngeal wall further away from the palate, making the pharynx abnormally deep (Arvystas & Shprintzen, 1984). When a deep pharynx is paired with a short palate (caused by clefting) that has decreased muscle bulk, the volume of the nasopharyngeal airway appears enormous (Figure 2–71).

## Severe Hypernasality

Hypernasal speech is reported in nearly 75% of children with VCFS, and when present, it is almost always severe. Hypernasality is considered separately from velopharyngeal insufficiency because the acoustic symptom does not necessarily correlate with the physical size of the velopharyngeal gap. In cases where there is absence of movement in the velopharyngeal valve, it is

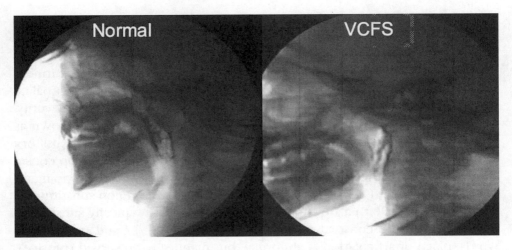

**FIGURE 2–71.** Structure of the nasopharynx and velopharyngeal valve in a normal (*left*) compared to an individual with VCFS, showing the increased volume of the pharynx in VCFS.

expected that hypernasality will be severe. In most cases of this type, articulation is severely impaired with ubiquitous glottal stop substitutions for nearly all sounds, even sounds that are not stop consonants (Video 2–17). It is known that there is a bidirectional correlation between VPI and glottal stop substitutions (Golding-Kushner, 2000; Henningsson & Isberg, 1991). In many cases of individuals with cleft palate who do not have VCFS, resolution of the compensatory glottal stop pattern of articulation will result in an improvement of movement in the velopharyngeal mechanism (Golding-Kushner, 2000; Henningsson & Isberg, 1991). However, this does not happen in VCFS (Golding-Kushner, 1991). Even with normal articulatory placement and production, almost all patients have gross VPI.

A more interesting phenomenon in VCFS is that even small velopharyngeal gaps often result in the perception of severe hypernasality (see the third case shown in Video 2–17). Most clinicians would intuitively suggest that small gaps result in mild hypernasal resonance. The reason for this apparent discrepancy is not known. One may hypothesize that the size of the nasal resonating chamber has something to do with it. Because the nasopharynx is very large, whatever sound leaks through even a small gap then has the opportunity to resonate in a large chamber above that site, and this is perceived as severe hypernasal resonance. The lack of correlation between velopharyngeal gap size during speech and the degree of perceived hypernasality is an important issue to understand in order to prevent the implementation of surgical procedures based solely on perceptual judgments of speech. It has been demonstrated that surgical outcomes are dependent on direct visual assessments of VPI (Shprintzen et al., 1979), not perceptual judgment. The goal of surgery is to eliminate the VPI by closing the gap completely.

## Severe Articulation Impairment (Glottal Stops)

Severe articulation impairment is found in more than 60% of children with VCFS (Golding-Kushner, 1991; Shprintzen, 1999). The articulation impairment in VCFS is not very different from that seen in other children with cleft palate in terms of type, but it is very different in terms of extent and severity. Children with VCFS develop patterns of articulation substitutions known as compensatory articulation. The most common component of compensatory articulation is a sound known as a glottal stop. A glottal stop is a stop consonant produced by the vocal cords (at the glottis) by closing and stopping air below the cords and then releasing it. Glottal stops are common substitutions in children with cleft palate and VPI. However, they are typically substituted only for other stop consonants, such as /p/, /b/, /t/, /d/, /k/, and /g/. In other words, place of articulation is abnormal, but manner is preserved (plosive). In children with VCFS, glottal stops are typically substituted for all consonant sounds, including stops, continuants, affricates, glides, and even nasals (Video 2–18). In order to understand how these sounds get established, it is necessary to know something about glottal stops.

Glottal stops are transcribed with the phonetic symbol /ʔ/. Most clinicians believe that glottal stops are not a sound in English and other languages such as French, Spanish, Italian, German, Greek, and others. This is not at all true. In fact, glottal stops are common sounds in all languages. However, they are not usually recognized as glottal stops or phonetically transcribed as glottal stops. For example, in the sentence, "I shot an arrow in the air," there are actually 5 glottal stop consonants. They are in the following locations:

ʔI shot ʔan ʔarrow ʔin the ʔair

In other words, each vowel that is not preceded by a pressure consonant sound like /p/, /b/, /t/, or /s/ has to be preceded by some form of stop consonant in order to build up enough pressure to start the vowel sound, because it is voiced and the vocal cords cannot vibrate without pressure being built up somewhere in the upper airway. Although the word "in" in that sentence might be transcribed as /ɪn/, it really should be transcribed as /ʔɪn/. Every time a sentence is started with a vowel, such as "I" or "A" or "An" or "Up" or "Inside," it is actually being started with a glottal stop. When babies begin to babble single "vowels" or repeated vowels, they are actually saying consonant-vowel-consonant utterances (CVC) or stringing together CVCs. If they say "oo," they are actually saying /ʔu/. If they say that perpetually cute "Uh-oh" that everyone seems to delight in hearing from babies, they are actually saying /ʔuʔo/. Glottal stop consonants also occur when there are rapid back to front consonant transitions that would be too difficult to articulate at normal rates of speech, such as the word "kitten." Very few people pronounce the *t* in kitten. Most people say /kɪʔɪn/.

Then how do glottal stops become established in VCFS and why for so many sounds? To explain how these sounds first become established, we need to look at how speech is developed and how speech is learned. The energy for speech production is provided by airflow from the lungs that passes between the vocal cords, an opening called the glottis, and into the upper airway (the vocal tract). The vocal tract contains a series of three regions that move in a coordinated way to modulate the airstream, controlling the direction and manner of airflow. The glottis is the first of these regions. The second is the velopharyngeal valve, which if open allows air to enter the nasal cavity and escape through the nose. This area is controlled by movement of the palate and pharyngeal walls, which need to contact each other to prevent air from entering the nasal cavity for speech that should normally be coming only out of the mouth. The third source of modulation includes the lips and tongue, which modify the shape of the oral cavity and which can make contact with the teeth, alveolar ridge, palate, and each other to create different consonant sounds. Vowels are produced with voice, meaning that the vocal cords vibrate while air passes through the glottis. Velopharyngeal movements occur to narrow the opening between the oral cavity and nasal cavity, but that movement may not close the opening between the mouth and nose completely. The lips and tongue change position according to the vowel being produced, but they do not contact each other, and there is no obstruction of the airstream that carries the sound. Vowels are generally learned correctly even in the presence of severe VPI. The nasal consonants /m/, /n/, and /ng/ (phonetically transcribed as ŋ) are produced when the lips or tongue obstruct the oral cavity while the velopharyngeal valve is open, permitting sound to come out of the nose. All other consonant sounds require impounding intraoral air pressure, which is only possible when velopharyngeal closure occurs to prevent air and the sound it carries from escaping through the nose. As pressure builds in the oral cavity, the lips and tongue are used to create an obstruction or constriction, which results in the production of various consonants. If the vocal cords vibrate at the same time as the lips and tongue are causing these constrictions, then the consonant is voiced. Voiced consonants in English are /m, n, ŋ, b, v, z, d, l, y, r, g/ (the hard g), /ʒ/ (the sound of the second g in *garage*), /dʒ/ (the sound of the *j* in *jay*), and /ð/ (the sound of the *th* in *this*). All of the voiceless sounds are consonants and include /s, f, h, k, t, p, ʃ/ (the *sh* sound in *shoe*), and /θ/ (the *th* sound in *think*). For these sounds, the vocal cords should be open, and the airstream travels into the oral cavity (there are no voiceless sounds that go to the nose), where it is shaped or stopped by the tongue and/or lips making contact with the oral structures.

Babies do not know how to make these sounds, but they do vocalize a lot. Crying is not shaped into speech, but at other times, babies randomly close their vocal cords while they are exhaling, which forces air through the cords to make voice. If the mouth is open, this sound will be interpreted as vowel-like cooing. If the lips are closed, it will sound like "mmm." A bit later on in development, as the baby's brain is beginning to myelinate and there is improved coordination, the baby will begin moving the palate and pharynx during these sounds, as well as the tongue and lips. During these random movements while sound is being produced, a /b/ or /g/ or /d/ may be produced. This marks the start of more diversified babbling. All of these sounds are initially produced purely by random movements. How do these get shaped into words? It is a perfect example of operant learning, as predicted by B. F. Skinner.

The learning process for speech starts with a trial and error. At some point, purely by random vocalizations, a baby will repeat a sound or sounds in the presence of a parent. Obviously, the sounds that are repeated the most are those that are the easiest for the child to make. The sound "ma" is a very common babbling sound in infants, and as babies get older, they naturally repeat sounds. At some point, the mother will be in close vicinity to the baby when "ma-ma" is uttered. As soon as it is heard, the mother will show great delight. The baby finds this to be reinforcing, and because the kisses and hugs came right after the baby said "ma-ma" the baby will be more likely to repeat the sound in the presence of her mother. That repetition will be reinforced over and over again until it is learned. It is not a mystery why the word or vernacular term for *mother* in essentially every language in the world has the /m/ sound in it. In English, commonly *mama*, or *mom*, or *mum*; in French, *maman*; in Norwegian, *mor*; in Hebrew, *ima*, and so son. This is because /m/ is the one of the earliest consonants produced, and the person in the environment of the child the most is mother. Similarly, the child may babble "ba-ba" in the presence of a bottle, the parent will attach the meaning to the utterance and reinforce the baby's utterance, and the baby will learn that what was reinforced means bottle. For babies with VCFS, babbling is severely restricted by the inability to produce pressure consonant sounds that require oral pressure, such as /p, b, t, d, s, z, g, k/, and so on. Because VPI prevents the proper production of the sound, there is no opportunity for caregivers to attach meaning to vocal attempts that may not even be recognized as attempts at those specific sounds. At some point, the child may randomly produce ʔaʔa. That repetition is similar to ba-ba in that the ʔ consonant is a stop pressure consonant. Place of articulation is different (the glottis rather than the lips), but a consonant is heard that distinguishes it from ma-ma and perhaps sounds close enough to da-da or pa-pa to be reinforced as a different word. What has happened is that the infant has produced a "pressure" consonant at a location in the system that can build air pressure before the air escapes through the velopharyngeal valve into the nasal cavity. The child therefore learns this substitution in a similar way for words like *go* or *ball* or *baby*. This is actually a clever solution to the problem of impounding air pressure for speech and is evidence of the drive to develop spoken language. The problem with it is that the same substitution is produced for all or nearly all consonants. In the early stages if speech development when reduplicated syllables are used for words, the glottal stop substitution works effectively, which is why the child learns it. However, as language development advances and utterances become longer, the glottal stop loses its effectiveness because everything sounds the same (Video 2–18). Consonants carry a significant amount of the meaning in language. Because all consonants sound the same for children with VCFS, their communication becomes unintelligible and ineffective in conveying meaning, limiting their expressive language or at least limiting the intelligibility of their communicative attempts. Therefore, although first words and the onset of language are often only slightly delayed in VCFS (Golding-Kushner et al., 1985), expressive language appears to be, and often is impaired. It is our experience that in many cases by the time the speech problem is recognized as a compensatory articulation pattern, the substitution pattern has become so deeply ingrained and generalized that, with the exception of nasal consonants /m/ and /n/, every other consonant has a compensatory substitution; sometimes glottal stops are even substituted for /m/ and /n/. Although a number of other compensations are also seen, including laryngeal fricatives, posterior nasal fricatives, and pharyngeal stops, the most frequent substitution by far for this group is the glottal stop.

Unfortunately, when speech is so severely impaired and unintelligible, clinicians often suspect that the child with VCFS is apraxic or dyspraxic. Although often diagnosed, dyspraxia is either not found in VCFS or at most is extremely rare. Most clinicians who do not have special training in speech patterns associated with cleft palate and VPI do not recognize glottal stops and think the pattern is one of consonant omissions. This is an easy error to make and the judgment is reinforced by the fact that the speakers producing glottal stops tend to produce very little lip, tongue, and facial movement because the sound is being made at the level of the larynx, eliminating the necessity to move the upper articulators. Failure to recognize glottal stops as a sound and therefore a sound substitution leads the clinician to believe that there is a motor planning problem (dyspraxia). Therapy approaches and the prognosis for treatment of dyspraxia are different from those for a compensatory articulation disorder. The articulation impairment typical of VCFS is almost always completely correctable. With rare exception, children with VCFS should have normal speech after appropriate therapy to correct the articulation errors and surgery to eliminate VPI.

### High Pitched Voice

High pitched voice is common in VCFS in childhood and occurs in more than half the cases based on clinical experience. There are several reasons why the voice would be high pitched, including a congenitally small larynx, laryngeal web that reduces the vibrating surface of the vocal cords, and small stature for age in early childhood, all of which can occur singly or in combination.

When children with VCFS eventually reach late adolescence and adulthood, vocal pitch normalizes, so understanding the natural history of this finding is important to avoid unnecessary treatment.

## Hoarseness

The frequency of hoarseness in VCFS is probably underestimated because speech and voice are disordered in so many different ways. If hypernasality is severe, it can sometimes mask hoarseness as a primary component of a communication impairment. Conversely, if hoarseness is very severe, it can sometimes mask hypernasal resonance if hypernasality is mild. It is probably true that a high percentage if not a majority of children with VCFS have some degree of hoarseness. In most cases it is mild and it does not result in aphonia. Hoarseness is typically caused by vocal cord anomalies, including asymmetry of the cords (Chegar et al., 2006) or laryngeal web. Hoarseness can also be secondary to chronic respiratory irritation from large tonsils, reactive airway disease, chronic coughing, or reflux. Although tonsillectomy and the treatment of airway symptoms and reflux may help to reduce or resolve hoarseness, it must also be kept in mind that a large number of children who do not have VCFS are hoarse, often from vocal abuse. In most cases, voice therapy is not indicated or difficult to implement.

## Language Impairment (Usually Mild Delay)

Language impairment is reported as a common problem in VCFS. It is true that the onset of speech and language is slightly delayed in most children with VCFS but in some cases the delay can be moderate to severe. It is uniformly reported that expressive language is more severely impaired than receptive (Golding-Kushner, 1991; Golding-Kushner, 2005; Golding-Kushner et al., 1985; Scherer et al., 1999). It is not yet known if the degree of language impairment is directly related to the degree of cognitive deficiency. It is also true that a percentage of children with VCFS qualify for the diagnosis of autism spectrum disorder (Antshel et al., 2006), and in these cases, language tends to be more significantly impaired. Scherer et al. (1999) found that language was more significantly impaired than other developmental milestones, although the specific reasons for the impairment could not be identified. In a review of 74 children with VCFS, Golding-Kushner (1991) found that there was no relationship between language delay and prevalence of glottal stop articulation pattern, and all but one of the VCFS subjects in her study who had normal language development had glottal stop patterns. At present, it is still not known if the degree of speech and language impairment or hypernasality is directly related to the degree of heart anomalies or other phenotypes. There are substantial data sets available that demonstrate the brain anatomy is abnormal in VCFS (Barnea-Goraly et al., 2003; Chow et al., 2002; Eliez et al., 2000; Kates et al., 2006), including reduced total brain volume. Therefore, it is certainly possible if not likely that language centers might be affected by the abnormal brain development. Current data sets that have reported specific language data have been small, and additional data are required to demonstrate the exact nature of language impairment.

## COGNITIVE, LEARNING, AND ATTENTIONAL DISORDERS

Cognitive, learning, intellectual, and attentional impairment are common in VCFS, occurring in nearly all cases. The issue of cognitive impairment is difficult to separate from overall behavioral and psychiatric disorders. It is recognized that individuals with schizophrenia and other psychiatric disorders have a significant deterioration of cognitive function and decreasing IQ scores. It has not yet been determined if the cognitive and behavioral problems associated with VCFS are interrelated or causally related. It is difficult to know how to categorize the various disorders in VCFS that stem from neuropsychological functioning. Because attention deficit disorder and autism spectrum disorder are so closely related to learning and academic achievement, we have grouped them with cognitive rather than psychiatric findings. Cognitive features of VCFS include:

159. Learning disabilities

160. Concrete thinking, difficulty with abstraction and problem solving

161. Low IQ

162. Drop in IQ scores in school years

163. Attention deficit hyperactivity disorder (ADD/ADHD)

164. Autism spectrum disorder (ASD)

### Learning Disabilities

Nearly all people with VCFS have learning problems to some extent. The two areas most relevant to school performance are difficulties with mathematics and reading comprehension. Although early letter and word recognition and rote reading skills are not significantly impaired in children with VCFS, their ability to extract meaning from what they read is. As reading becomes more complex, reading comprehension becomes more difficult. These types of problems with reading usually become most apparent in second or third grade when reading tasks are more likely to encompass more complex sentences and longer pieces of literature. Extracting meaning from simple sentences and phrases is not problematic, but complex sentences and paragraphs present challenges for children with VCFS, especially if the message in the writing is abstract or figurative or if there is use of metaphors or similes. While a child with VCFS will be able to extract meaning from the simple sentence, "I saw Jack," the same child may have a hard time decoding "Jack and Jill went up the hill to fetch a pail of water." The sentence is complex with multiple nouns related to the action verb. Similarly, the sentence, "The ocean roared like a lion warning its enemy to stay away," would be extremely difficult for a child with VCFS to interpret because of the allusion to a lion that clearly has nothing to do with the ocean in the eyes of the child. The sentence might even cause the child with VCFS to worry about lions being in the vicinity of the ocean because the child will interpret the sentence concretely, believing that the ocean and the lion go together.

Mathematics presents similar problems. The early learning of numbers and simple arithmetic is not significantly impaired in children with VCFS. Learning simple mathematic functions or problems of addition or subtraction with rote memory is a skill that is often mastered with relative ease by children with VCFS. However, once an attempt is made to teach the functions of mathematics, the concepts of mathematics, and the theory of mathematical functions, the typical child with VCFS has enormous problems. A simple example is as follows. A first grader with VCFS is taught the problem, $3 + 2 = 5$. After several repetitions, the problem is learned and learned permanently. The teacher then attempts to teach the child about addition, stating that in addition, it does not matter what side of the $+$ the numbers (the addends) are. The sum is always the same. The teacher then asks the child, "If $3 + 2 = 5$, then what does $2 + 3$ equal?" The child with VCFS will be lost. In order for the child to learn what $2 + 3$ equals, the problem will need to be taught the problem as a second separate and distinct equation, not as a mathematical concept.

## Concrete Thinking, Difficulty with Abstraction and Problem Solving

The primary problem in cognitive function in people with VCFS is a significant deficiency in executive functioning. Executive functioning is seated in the prefrontal cortex, an area of the brain known to be smaller than normal in VCFS (Eliez et al., 2000; Kates et al., 2004). Executive functioning is the portion of our cognitive and mental capacity that includes problem solving and the ability to be flexible in our thinking and allows us to direct our cognitive abilities towards a goal. Executive functioning also allows us to use our cognitive faculties to control impulses and emotional responses, focus our attention, and apply lessons we have learned from current planning and behavior towards future planning and behavior. All of these cognitive skills controlled by executive functioning are impaired in VCFS and cut across both cognitive and mental capacities. The inability to plan things out "in your head" results in difficulty with problem solving. Moreover, people with VCFS interpret everything in a very literal and concrete way. It is sometimes difficult to determine exactly what children with VCFS are describing about what they think or feel because they cannot grasp the typical abstract terms others use. "Feeling blue" or "hot under the collar" would not be learned in anything other than a concrete way, relating to color in the first case and temperature in the second. It is sometimes difficult in children with VCFS to figure out what they are referring to when they say they are hearing voices. Sometimes they are referring to hearing themselves think, and they interpret this as hearing a voice in their heads. Obviously, it can be quite scary to think that your child is hearing voices, but the situation may not be as serious as it sounds if it simply refers to a literal description of what they are "hearing."

Another example can be used to demonstrate this problem. The story involves a patient who lived in New York City, in the Bronx, who was 17 years old. She asked her father if she could go to visit her grandmother in Brooklyn, a long subway ride from her family's apartment. Although a long subway ride (nearly an hour) and the need to change trains once, the connection was not complicated. Her father, who worked for the transit system, described for her how to make the trip in detail. He told her that the ride was easy because both their apartment in the Bronx and her grandmother's apartment in Brooklyn were at the end of the subway line. He told her to walk out of their apartment and that she would see the steps up to the subway platform straight ahead. He told her to walk up the steps, put a token in any of the entrance gates, and to turn to the left and walk up the next flight of steps. This would put her on the departing side of the train tracks and she could walk into any subway car with an open door that had the number 6 in a green circle in the window. He told her to sit facing a window so she could see the station signs as the train entered the platform for each stop. He told her that when she saw "Bleeker Street" to get off of the train and to walk straight ahead following the sign that had an orange circle with the letter D in the middle of it that said, "Downtown and Brooklyn." She would then get on any train at that platform that had a D in an orange circle on the window that also said "Coney Island" on the sign in the window. This was the end of the line. He told her to exit the subway car and turn left to walk to the end of the platform where there was a stairway down to the street. He told her that when she came down the stairs that her grandmother's apartment was directly across the street and gave her the number of the building and where she would see the number, telling her how to get into the building by ringing the buzzer. The young lady wrote down the directions, but also committed them to memory and was fine going to Brooklyn and did not get lost. Unfortunately, she did get lost coming home. How did she fail to negotiate the return trip? Because when she asked how to get home, her father told her, "It's simple…just do the opposite." Opposite is one of those concepts that require executive functioning to figure out the problem and use both temporal and spatial imagery to apply the solution. What he needed to do was to give her the directions for the return trip exactly as he had given her the directions going.

## Low IQ

IQ scores are the numbers that are used to categorize someone as having normal, superior, or below normal (retarded) intellect. In general, IQ scores measured by standardized tests like the Wechsler Intelligence Scales (for children or adults) use the standard of 100 as average. On this test and others like it, the range of IQ scores from 90 to 110 is labeled Average. A score of 110 to 120 is High Average, and 121 to 130 is Superior. Above 131 is Very Superior. Scores from 80 to 89 are Low Average, and 70 to 79 is Borderline. Below 70 is Extremely Low and in the past carried the label "mental retardation." IQ scores are generally considered to be good predictors of performance in school and later in life in terms of capabilities to live an independent life. A number of studies have been done that have measured IQ scores in VCFS (Antshel, Abdul Sabur, Roizen, Fremont, & Kates, 2005; Golding-Kushner et al., 1985; Moss et al., 1999; Swillen et al., 1997) and typically put the mean IQ for VCFS in the borderline range between 70 and 80. There is often a discrepancy of 10 points or more between verbal (higher) and performance (lower) IQ scores, but this is not universal in VCFS (Kates et al., 2005). The mean IQ score in the borderline range means that there are a substantial number of individuals with VCFS who have IQ scores in the normal range, and others who are below 70 with some being substantially below 70. Our own data indicate a wide range of variability of IQ scores in VCFS, with some in the superior range, and some individuals with very low IQ scores. In many cases, we have found that IQ is not always predictive of school performance, especially when there is a discrepancy between verbal and performance IQ.

## Drop in IQ Scores in School Years

It was first noted in 1985 that IQ scores were higher for younger children with VCFS than older children (Golding-Kushner et al., 1985). It was suggested that the decrease in scores that was observed using cross-sectional data was related to differences in the nature of the tests used with younger versus older children, and the lack of development of abstract reasoning skills by the time it would be expected to have occurred. The tests for older children rely more on language-based tasks and abstract thinking that would be expected to have developed and matured. It was not thought that there was any loss of ability or skill that had been previously established. Our experience now, based on both cross-sectional and longitudinal data, is that a decrease in IQ scores does not happen for all people with VCFS, but it does occur for some. It is not clear if those who experience the decrease are individuals who are most likely to develop mental illness or if this simply reflects a specific type of learning deficit that makes some individuals with VCFS compare more poorly to their peers over time. There is no strong evidence to suggest that the decline represents a deterioration of cognitive abilities rather than a comparative problem. Because IQ scores are comparative scores, meaning that they are based on the performance of that individual in relation to a large cohort of individuals who are the same chronological age, it is possible that cognitive abilities do not deteriorate but simply do not progress as rapidly as others' in the same age range. It is also possible that the nature of IQ tests makes them a less accurate measure of the strengths of individuals with VCFS. Portions of IQ tests are timed, almost always a problem for children with VCFS, and some portions tend to highlight the difficulties with abstraction and problem solving that are the basic substance of VCFS learning disorders. As more longitudinal studies are completed, the nature of these shifts in IQ score will become elucidated.

## Attention Deficit Hyperactivity Disorder (ADD/ADHD)

Attention deficit hyperactivity disorder is a very common finding in VCFS, and a number of studies have demonstrated the prevalence of ADD/ADHD to be high. Antshel et al. (2006) found 42.8% of a sample of 84 children with VCFS met DSM-IV (APA, 2004) diagnostic criteria for ADD/ADHD. Unlike the general population and a control sample in the same study, there was no difference in the frequency of ADD/ADHD in males and females with VCFS, although in the general population and the control sample, males outnumbered females. Of those subjects with VCFS who had ADD/ADHD, the largest number had the inattentive subtype. These numbers are very similar to those reported by Feinstein et al. (2002) and Gothelf et al. (2004), who found ADD/ADHD in 46.4% of 28 subjects with VCFS and 41.2% of 58 subjects, respectively. This close agreement on the frequency of VCFS in three different populations, including one from Israel (the Gothelf study) and one from California (the Feinstein study) and a third made up of subjects from all over the United States and Western Europe (Antshel et al., 2006), clearly demonstrates a solid predisposition to ADD/ADHD in children with VCFS. As longitudinal data are collected, the natural history of ADD/ADHD and its relationship with other psychiatric diagnoses will become clearer.

## Autism Spectrum Disorder (ASD)

The occurrence of ASD in the VCFS population is a matter of significant controversy. Vorstman et al. (2006) reported that 50% of a sample of 60 children with VCFS met the criteria for ASD. The age range of the sample was birth to 20 years. The article received a published response from Eliez (2007), who argued that the overlap in symptoms typically associated with ASD and those found in children with VCFS does not necessarily imply that children with VCFS have a high frequency of ASD. He warned that applying the term "autistic" to children with VCFS could lead to treatment errors, especially in relation to behavioral and psychiatric disorders. A second report also found a high rate of diagnosis of ASD in a sample of 40 children with VCFS (Antshel et al.,

2006). Antshel et al. reported that 42% of the sample met diagnostic criteria for ASD, while 20% of the total sample met strict criteria for autism. Could it be that autism has been a clinical feature of VCFS for all of these years and no one has noticed? Why did it take more than 30 years for clinicians and scientists to realize that autism or ASD was a clinical feature of VCFS, and even before that, of DiGeorge syndrome, conotruncal anomalies face syndrome, and Sedláčková syndrome? There are several possibilities.

The first possibility is that the features of VCFS (under its many names) have not changed at all, but the definition of ASD has. This is, of course, true. Although autism has been recognized for more than 60 years, ASD as a diagnostic term is relatively new. The term autism was originally coined in 1910 by Bleuler (Wolff, 2004), but as a specific disorder, Kanner is typically given credit for describing the condition and spawning both interest and research (Kanner, 1943). Kanner described the clinical features of autism as "extreme autistic aloneness," poor language usage that prevented effective communication, repetitive behaviors (such as arm flapping), and a constant effort to keep things consistently the same that had an obsessive quality. This classical form of autism was always easy to recognize clinically because of distinctly bizarre patterns of behavior and the avoidance of human contact that was less social and seemed to be an indication of extreme discomfort. It is of interest to note that Kanner thought that autism was a rare disorder, a far cry from today's statistics that tout prevalence statistics in the range of 1:150 according to Center for Disease Control's Autism and Developmental Disabilities Monitoring (Center for Disease Control and Prevention, 2007). A prevalence this high (nearly 1% of the general population) seems a remarkably large number at face value. It can only be explained by an expansion of the criteria for the diagnosis of autism. In more recent years, a number of other disorders have been interpreted as being milder expressions of autism. Initially known as *pervasive developmental delay* (PDD), the spectrum of disorders that has sprouted from the original delineation of autism is now known as ASD and includes:

1. **Autism**.

2. **Asperger syndrome**—a developmental disorder marked by repetitive routines, odd speech and language patterns, poor social skills, and bizarre preoccupations, but without the cognitive impairment that is often found in autism.

3. **Childhood disintegrative disorder (CDD)**—this extremely rare disorder occurs almost exclusively in males and probably has a population prevalence of approximately 1:50,000. Children with CDD develop normally until 4 or 5 years of age, and then there is a rapid disintegration of function, including loss of vocabulary and language, degradation of intellect and motor abilities, and severe behavioral abnormalities.

4. **Rett syndrome**—a rare disorder with a population prevalence of approximately 1:15,000 that occurs almost exclusively in females and is

characterized by a marked degradation of cognitive and mental abilities in infants and toddlers to a severe type of autistic behavior. A genetic link to Rett syndrome has been identified, one that does not occur in children with other forms of ASD. A candidate gene, *MECP2*, has been identified on the X chromosome, and it seems that the syndrome is only expressed in girls because males who have the mutation do not survive; this is because they only have one X chromosome and the Y chromosome does not have a corresponding gene to counteract the mutated version.

5. **PDD-Not Otherwise Specified (PDD-NOS)**—although this term is confusing, it is a firm diagnosis listed in the DSM manual and is a milder form of autism.

This somewhat involved description points out that the high prevalence of ASD is because the diagnostic umbrella has expanded so that 1:150 children is standing in its shadow. As more and more people fall under the ASD umbrella, the overlap between the symptoms of ASD and VCFS becomes larger. Put another way, the more symptoms that are listed as features of ASD, and the more symptoms that are listed as behavioral components of VCFS, the greater the chance for a match. Because diagnostic inventories and standardized tests function as categorical probability scales (i.e., if you have this, that, and the other thing, you have the disease), the larger the number of opportunities to endorse individual symptoms, the higher the probability that you have the disease. An analogy would be as follows. In order to determine if someone has a cold, you have to endorse the following symptoms: stuffy nose, cough, sneezing, and serous otitis media. But people who have allergic rhinitis will endorse all of those symptoms. So will people with influenza. So will people with the early stages of chicken pox. There is no doubt that people with allergies, the flu, and chicken pox do not have colds, but they endorse the same symptoms. This may be why children with VCFS are often diagnosed with autism or ASD. Are there children with VCFS who are autistic? Yes. Clinical experience has shown that there are some but not many children with VCFS who are indistinguishable from other children with autism. It is not, however, half or even nearly half of children with VCFS. Although a probability score may qualify some children with VCFS for the diagnosis of ASD, the question is whether qualitatively they resemble other children with ASD who do not have VCFS.

## PSYCHIATRIC DISORDERS

The first report of psychiatric illness as a clinical finding in VCFS was in 1992 (Shprintzen et al., 1992). This report was actually a brief letter to the editor of the *American Journal of Medical Genetics* with a description of individuals with VCFS who had been seen initially as young children in the 1970s and treated for various problems, including hypernasal speech, heart disease, and learning problems. When their referring problems had been resolved, they were either discharged from care or not given routine follow-up appointments. Years later, we were contacted by their parents with reports of psychiatric illness. Twelve of the 90 cases we were following at the time reported psychiatric problems, with the majority diagnosed as chronic schizophrenia with paranoid delusions. The age of onset ranged from 10 years to 21 years, with the average age of onset 14 years. Although not reported at the time, the median age of the sample was 16, with a bimodal distribution with the peaks at 15 and 19 years of age. The co-occurrence of the report of psychosis in VCFS in 1992 with the discovery that the syndrome was caused by a microdeletion from chromosome 22 (Scambler et al., 1992) launched extensive study of VCFS because of the potential that 22q11.2 housed a strong genetic link to schizophrenia. Since that initial publication, many researchers have published reports of findings that psychiatric disorders are common in VCFS (Antshel et al., 2006; Baker & Skuse, 2005; Bassett et al., 2003; Feinstein et al., 2002; Murphy, Jones, & Owen, 1999; Papolos et al., 1996; Pulver et al., 1994; Usiskin et al., 1999). The reported rate of psychosis associated with VCFS has ranged from approximately 10 to 32%, with a wide variety of ascertainment sources probably accounting for the differences (Baker & Skuse, 2005; Bassett et al., 2003; Feinstein et al., 2002; Murphy et al., 1999; Papolos et al., 1996; Pulver et al., 1994; Usiskin et al., 1999). The true prevalence of psychosis may be difficult to calculate in VCFS because individuals with the mildest expression of the syndrome may not come to attention and be diagnosed and therefore never be accessible to research. Conversely, it is known that individuals with VCFS exist among the population of people with psychosis who may not have been diagnosed with VCFS (Horowitz, Shifman, Rivlin, Pisanté, & Darvasi, 2005; Karayiorgou et al., 1995). Although an exact prevalence of psychiatric illness among all people with VCFS cannot be known, it is clearly much higher than in the general population, and most researchers regard VCFS to be the most significant genetic risk for psychosis in general and schizophrenia specifically, with a risk that could be as much as 25 times higher than the general population.

There is also some controversy regarding the nature of the psychiatric illness found in VCFS. Both schizophrenia (Murphy et al., 1999) and bipolar disorder (Papolos et al., 1996) have been reported to occur in people with VCFS, and it has also been suggested that the mental illness associated with VCFS is not either of those entities, but rather a psychiatric phenotype specific to VCFS (Verhoeven, Tuinier, & Curfs, 2000). In part, this controversy is an artificial one if it is inspired by the notion that schizophrenia, bipolar disorder, schizoaffective disorder, and other psychotic conditions are separate and distinct diseases rather than symptoms of a more general process that causes psychosis. Psychiatric symptoms associated with VCFS include:

165. Schizophrenia

166. Bipolar disorder

167. Rapid or ultrarapid cycling of mood disorder

168. Mood disorder, dysthymia, cyclothymia

169. Depression

170. Hypomania

171. Manic depressive psychosis

172. Schizoaffective disorder

173. Impulsiveness

174. Flat affect

175. Social immaturity

176. Obsessive-compulsive disorder

177. Generalized anxiety disorder

178. Phobias

179. Severe startle response

180. Separation anxiety

## Schizophrenia

In the first report of psychiatric illness in VCFS, Shprintzen et al. (1992) reported a substantial prevalence of schizophrenia in VCFS. Subsequent studies have also reported that schizophrenia is a feature of VCFS (Bassett et al., 2003; Horowitz et al., 2005; Karayiorgou et al., 1995; Murphy et al., 1999; Pulver et al., 1994). Schizophrenia has a population prevalence of approximately 1%, meaning that VCFS has at least a 25 if not 30 times higher frequency than the general population, and this indicates the importance of studying VCFS. Clearly, the implication is that something in the deleted region of 22q11.2 protects people from schizophrenia or other mental illness, so when the deletion occurs, that protection is missing and the disease develops.

Schizophrenia is defined symptomatically, as are most psychiatric disorders. People with schizophrenia cannot distinguish between what is real and what is not real. They may hear voices or have visual hallucinations, or they may believe that other people are hearing their thoughts or reading their minds. Their thoughts and behaviors are unpredictable and disorganized, and this can often evoke fear in people around them. Many of these symptoms do occur in people with VCFS. Part of the challenge in interpreting these findings in VCFS is that they depend on descriptions from the person who has them. Because of their concreteness, people with VCFS may have a difficult time explaining what they are feeling internally. That being said, there is no doubt that schizophrenia is a part of the VCFS phenotype.

An interesting phenomenon observed as a clinician is that of all of the findings associated with VCFS, this is the one that distresses parents the most. Even for babies born with severe congenital heart disease, the issue that parents seem most worried about is mental illness and, within that realm, schizophrenia. Having had contact with thousands of patients, a discernible pattern regarding the concern about mental illness is obvious. Families come in with infants with tetralogy of Fallot or interrupted aortic arch, pulmonary atresia, large VSDs, and other major heart anomalies who have had a positive FISH study. Anyone who has a computer immediately goes on-line and reads about VCFS. On some Web sites, and in chatlines and listservs, they read about mental illness and its consequences. It is an interesting phenomenon that there are bigger concerns over quality of life problems than quantity of life problems. At the research end of the equation, this may explain why the largest amount of research activity associated with VCFS has been in the psychiatric realm.

## Bipolar Disorder

This category includes rapid or ultrarapid cycling of mood, mood disorder, dysthymia, cyclothymia, depression, hypomania, and manic depressive psychosis. Although the initial reports describing psychosis in VCFS focused on schizophrenia, another study suggested that the mental illness seen in VCFS is actually in the bipolar spectrum, and that children with VCFS have childhood bipolar disorder (Papolos et al., 1996). Some clinicians classify bipolar disorder according to symptom presentation. Cases are classified as bipolar I or bipolar II depending on presenting symptoms. Bipolar I disorder (BP I or bipolar type I) is the more common of the two and is diagnosed when there are recurrent episodes of mania and depression. Bipolar II (BP II or bipolar type II) differs from BP I in that the episodes of elevated mood are *hypomanic* rather than manic, meaning that they are not as severe as seen in BP I. It is during severe manic episodes that psychosis often develops, a condition that was previously labeled as manic depressive psychosis before clinicians adopted the term bipolar disorder. Childhood bipolar disorder is a diagnosis that is very controversial, and not everyone believes that it represents an actual psychiatric diagnosis. Scientists who study childhood bipolar disorder indicate that the symptoms often mimic ADD/ADHD. Mood shifts, known as dysthymia and cyclothymia, can occur in association with childhood bipolar disorder. Dysthymia is a depressed mood, typically lasting longer than a major depressive episode but not as severe in terms of the depth of the depression. Cyclothymia is on the bipolar II spectrum of disorders and is diagnosed if the person with dysthymia has at least one episode of hypomania. Hypomania is an elevated or irritable mood that is not as severe as a full manic episode and has no evidence of psychosis. The most severe form of the mood disorder that accompanies childhood bipolar disorder in relation to mood swings is the rapid cycling or ultrarapid cycling variant. Whereas most people with bipolar disorder have cycles of mood changes that last for weeks or months, children with rapid or ultrarapid cycling shift moods several times a day, or even several times in an hour. This type of bipolar disorder was reported to occur in VCFS by Papolos et al. (1996). In fact, Papolos reported all types of bipolar disorder associated with VCFS in a series of 25 cases of VCFS. A recent study (Aneja et al., 2007) reported that the frequency of mania in VCFS does not vary significantly from the frequency of mania in nonsyndromic children who have ADD/ADHD, but that the presence of mania in VCFS may have other implications for the presence of psychiatric problems than in the general population.

Although not all clinicians and scientists agree with the bipolar diagnosis in children, mood disorders have been reported widely in children with VCFS. The confusion is compounded by the treatment of the disorder. Positive responses have been seen in some children by giving them mood stabilizers, including drugs like valproic acid (divalproex sodium, brand name Depakote), lamotrigine (brand name Lamictal), and oxcarbazepine (Trileptal). These drugs were developed and marketed originally as anticonvulsants but were subsequently found to have positive effects on bipolar disorder with respect to mood stabilization. Successful outcomes have been observed clinically in treating children and adults with VCFS with these medications, but only in carefully selected cases. Conversely, patients have also selectively responded to other types of medications, including antipsychotics, atypical antipsychotics, and even antihypertensives (Graf et al., 2001; O'Hanlon, Ritchie, Smith, & Patel, 2003).

One caveat that needs to be mentioned is that people with VCFS also have a high prevalence of thyroid disorders that can also cause problems that resemble bipolar symptoms. Lethargy, flat affect, low energy, and poor attention are all possible symptoms of hypothyroidism.

## Schizoaffective Disorder

Schizoaffective disorder is a clinical presentation with symptoms of bipolar disorder (mania, depression) but with symptoms that also meet the criteria for schizophrenia and psychosis. People with schizoaffective disorder are often treated with both mood stabilizers and antipsychotics. Two of the subjects with VCFS reported by Papolos et al. (1996) were diagnosed with schizoaffective disorder.

## Impulsiveness

Impulsiveness, or poor impulse control, is a common finding in VCFS. It is probably true that nearly all children with VCFS have some degree of impulsivity. Although there are standardized diagnostic criteria for impulsivity and not all people with VCFS will meet them, it is basically true that people with

VCFS are generally poor at controlling impulses to some extent. Impulsivity is a common finding in people with ADD/ADHD and bipolar disorder (especially in hypomanic or manic phases). However, it is also true that the problems with executive functioning contribute to impulsivity, because people with VCFS have a difficult time determining the outcomes of their behavior in a time-deferred manner.

## Flat Affect

Flat affect is also a common finding in VCFS, even when not accompanied by other psychiatric diagnoses, and was one of the first behavioral characteristics reported (Golding-Kushner et al., 1985). Children with VCFS are often shy and clingy. Because they tend to avoid unfamiliar situations, their response when exposed to something new or unfamiliar is to withdraw. It is also possible that early communication impairments and poor social experiences tend to make them withdraw. At this point, no link has been made between early flat affect and subsequent psychiatric disorders.

## Social Immaturity

Social immaturity should not be a surprise in children with VCFS. The overall developmental delay that occurs in nearly all cases of VCFS is also seen in delayed maturation of social skills, play, and motor milestones that lag behind their peers. The gaps in early childhood tend to be relatively small because most play in toddlers and young children is not particularly sophisticated or language dependent. With advancing age, especially in late childhood and adolescence, play becomes increasingly dependent on language, imagination, problem solving, and other aspects of executive functioning. Early teen years can be a departure point where children with VCFS begin to separate from early childhood playmates.

## Obsessive-Compulsive Disorder

Reports of the frequency of obsessive-compulsive disorder (OCD) in VCFS vary from under 5% (Antshel et al., 2006) to approximately 25% of cases (Gothelf et al., 2004). This difference may be a critical one because the presence of OCD in combination with a specific COMT genotype (presence of the *COMT^{met}* allele on the nondeleted copy of chromosome 22) has been reported to be a risk factor for the development of schizophrenia in VCFS (Gothelf et al., 2007). An earlier report (Papolos et al., 1996) reported the frequency of OCD at 8%.

### Generalized Anxiety Disorder

Generalized anxiety is the presence of chronic anxiety when there are no apparent provoking stimuli. The reported range of the frequency of generalized anxiety disorder in VCFS is nearly 20% (Antshel et al., 2006) to 28% (Feinstein et al., 2002), although anxiety disorders in general (including OCD, phobias, separation anxiety, etc.) occur in more than 60% of cases. Generalized anxiety is more debilitating in the sense that it is not stimulus specific and nearly anything may cause an anxiety response. Very often, parents and others respond to anxiety by calling attention to it, punishing it, or trying to calm their children down, all of which tend to induce additional anxiety. It is also important to stress for parents that this problem is not the child's fault and it is not something the child is doing on purpose. Anxiety is a true physiologic response, with heightened sensitivity of the autonomic nervous system resulting in a number of observable reactions, including perspiration, rapid heartbeat, increased blood pressure, and a slowdown in the digestive system. When in a heightened state of arousal, any additional stress tends to be very disorganizing and may prompt severe emotional responses. Some children are helped by maintaining a calm environment and relaxation techniques; others respond to professional attention, medication, or both.

### Phobias

Phobias are another clinical symptom associated with anxiety and are common in VCFS. A frequency of approximately one quarter of individuals with VCFS has been reported (Antshel et al., 2006), although Feinstein et al. (2002) reported a prevalence of 60% for specific phobias in their sample. A common phobia in VCFS is thunder and other loud noises. This, together with the next clinical finding, a severe startle response, has led some clinicians to question if children with VCFS have hyperacusis and a sensitivity to loud noises. They do not.

### Severe Startle Response

Children with VCFS may also have a severe startle response, especially to loud noises, but to other surprising stimuli as well. This would be expected in cases where there was generalized anxiety disorder, because the autonomic nervous system is already in a state of arousal. It does not take much under these circumstances to cause a dramatic startle response. The addition of a loud, sudden stimulus would certainly initiate a strong response that would have a disorganizing effect on the child.

## Separation Anxiety

Separation anxiety is common in VCFS and is regarded as a possible warning sign for the development of childhood bipolar disorder (Papolos et al., 1996). Feinstein et al. (2002) reported a frequency of just over 20% in their sample of 28 children with VCFS. The long-term significance of separation anxiety has not been confirmed as yet, but because it is one of the earliest observations of abnormal emotional response, it is likely an important attribute to study.

# MISCELLANEOUS ANOMALIES

With 180 anomalies listed above, we are nearing the end of the list of anomalies that are clinical features of VCFS, but there are still 10 more. A number of miscellaneous problems, some rare, are perplexing and potentially dangerous. They include:

181. Thrombocytopenia

182. Bernard-Soulier syndrome

183. Juvenile rheumatoid arthritis

184. Poor temperature regulation

185. Spontaneous oxygen desaturation without apnea

186. Vasomotor instability

## Thrombocytopenia

Thrombocytopenia, a low platelet count, is a common finding in VCFS, although in most cases it is not present in childhood. As the child with VCFS reaches adolescence and puberty, the platelet count begins to fall, often to borderline or slightly low levels. In VCFS, the platelet problem is caused by the deletion of one copy of the gene *GP1Bß* that resides in the 22q11.2 region deleted in VCFS. *GP1Bß* is responsible for forming a glycoprotein on the surface of platelet cells. Deficiency or abnormality of this glycoprotein results in giant platelets and the potential for delayed clotting time. The surface protein mediated by *GP1Bß* causes the platelets to adhere to the surfaces of wound sites, thus beginning the clotting process. In most cases, the mild thrombocytopenia associated with the deletion does not cause excessive bleeding problems, but in some cases, as will be discussed next in relation to Bernard-Soulier syndrome, there can be serious consequences. It is recommended that children with VCFS have a platelet analysis every year with their well-child examination.

## Bernard-Soulier Syndrome

Bernard-Soulier syndrome is a bleeding disorder caused by a number of different platelet surface protein abnormalities, which include the *GP1Bß* that resides in the normally deleted region on chromosome 22, the cause of VCFS. Bernard-Soulier is characterized by bruising, prolonged bleeding time with delayed clotting, hemorrhages, and severe bleeding during periods in females. One form of Bernard-Soulier is an autosomal recessive disorder caused by a mutation in *GP1Bß*. With this specific mutation, it would normally take two copies of the mutant gene to result in the disorder. People with one copy of the mutant gene and one copy of the normal gene would not have a bleeding disorder. The mutant gene occurs infrequently in the general population. People who have VCFS are missing one copy of *GP1Bß*. If the remaining copy is not the mutant copy but a normally functioning gene, they will not have a bleeding disorder, although they may show mild effects of reduced gene activity because only one copy is present. However, if the single copy they have is the mutant allele, there is no normal gene on the other copy of chromosome 22 to counteract the mutant gene. In this situation the mutant gene will therefore be expressed. In other words, the deletion unmasks a recessive mutation in much the same way that X-linked recessive disorders are expressed in males because of the absence of a second X chromosome. This unmasking of a recessive gene has been reported in VCFS (Budarf et al., 1995; Ludlow et al., 1996) and, although rare, it is a finding in VCFS related to the deletion.

## Juvenile Rheumatoid Arthritis

Juvenile rheumatoid arthritis (JRA) has been reported as a rare finding in VCFS, but it has been reported as a feature of the syndrome (Rasmussen, Williams, & Ayoub, 1996; Sullivan et al., 1997; Verloes et al., 1998). The cause of JRA in individuals with VCFS is unknown, but it is one of a number of autoimmune problems that may be related to abnormalities of the immune system (Sullivan et al., 1997; Verloes et al., 1998). The number of reported cases of JRA in people with VCFS is small at this time, but a population-based study of chromosome rearrangements and the frequency of JRA and other immune disorders has demonstrated that the occurrence of JRA in VCFS is clearly a syndromic feature (Bache, Nielsen, Rostgaard, Tommerup, & Frisch, 2007).

## Poor Temperature Regulation

Clinical experience has revealed that a number of people with VCFS have difficulty with body temperature regulation. We have noted a number of cases where body temperature fluctuated dramatically in the absence of other symptoms that might signal the presence of a viral or bacterial infection. In a small number of cases, we have documented core temperatures that were very low, below 35°C. It is possible that these abnormal temperatures are related to poor circulation or idiosyncratic responses of the blood vessels in terms of constriction and dilation. It is also possible that the temperature regulation center of the brain, the hypothalamus, is anomalous. It is also possible that abnormal thyroid function plays a role. This phenomenon may not be common in VCFS, but this is not known and there have been no controlled studies to assess this problem.

### Spontaneous Oxygen Desaturation without Apnea

A number of cases have been observed who have had spontaneous and precipitous drops in arterial oxygen saturation that were not prompted by obstructive or central apneic episodes or cardiovascular events. The explanation for this observation while patients were being closely monitored by pulse oximetry is unknown. It is possible that this may represent some type of unusual vascular response similar to Reynaud's phenomenon. Pulse oximetry reads oxygen saturation by analyzing the color of the blood based on the absorption of light wavelengths by hemoglobin. Therefore, pulse oximeters are confounded by venous congestion and reduced peripheral blood flow, both of which are common phenomena in VCFS. It is therefore possible that pulse oximetry may *read* decreased oxygen saturation but that the reading is a false positive and related only to the location where the probe is placed, typically a finger, toe, or earlobe.

### Vasomotor Instability

Vasomotor instability is a term typically associated with perimenopausal women who experience "hot flashes." In its more severe form, it can be a dangerous and life-threatening condition resulting in severe drop in blood pressure, loss of consciousness, and abnormal heart rhythms. Several neonates with VCFS have had severe vasomotor instability following heart surgery. The success rate with heart surgery in VCFS is very similar to that seen in the children with the same heart anomalies who do not have VCFS (Anaclerio et al., 2004), and it is therefore likely that this abnormal response of the autonomic nervous system is unusual.

## SECONDARY DEVELOPMENTAL SEQUENCES

Sequences (see Chapter 1, Box 1) are recurring groupings of symptoms that are etiologically heterogeneous, although many are strongly associated with known syndromes that have firm identifiable causes. For example, Robin sequence (the association of micrognathia, U-shaped cleft palate, and upper airway obstruction) is one of the most common developmental sequences and is strongly associated with Stickler syndrome, which is caused by a mutation in a collagen-forming gene. Approximately one third of cases of Robin sequence have Stickler syndrome (Shprintzen, 1988; Shprintzen & Singer, 1992). The second most common syndromic cause of Robin sequence is VCFS (Shprintzen, 1988; Shprintzen & Singer, 1992) and has no relation to collagen abnormalities. The presence of secondary sequences is often confusing. Because the names of these secondary sequences are familiar and have been confused with syndromes, some people believe that the assignation of the label Robin or DiGeorge or holoprosencephaly excludes other diagnoses or the presence of other syndromes. The opposite is actually true. The presence of a developmental sequence almost always signals the presence of a more definitive syndromic diagnosis. The anomalies in VCFS trigger a number of developmental sequences, including:

187. Robin sequence

188. DiGeorge sequence

189. Potter sequence

190. Holoprosencephaly

## Robin Sequence

Robin sequence is caused by a mandible that is of abnormal size or in an abnormal position during embryogenesis, which prevents the tongue from descending from the skull base, where it normally sits at approximately 9 weeks following fertilization. The palatal shelves sit vertically alongside the tongue before it descends in the oral cavity. Once the tongue is out of the way of the palatal shelves, they flip into a horizontal orientation, grow towards the midline, and fuse. If the mandible does not grow sufficiently to make room for the tongue to descend, the palatal shelves cannot fuse because of the physical obstacle of the tongue in the midline. After birth, the abnormal mandible also causes airway obstruction. Babies, normally nasal breathers, attempt to breathe with their mouths closed, but the tongue sits posteriorly in a position that obstructs the airway. The triad of findings is therefore all caused by the abnormal mandible. Mandibular abnormalities that can lead to Robin sequence may be categorized as micrognathia (small mandible), retrognathia (retropositioned mandible), or microretrognathia (a small mandible that is also retropositioned), as discussed by Cohen (1999). In VCFS, the mandible is structurally normal but retropositioned because of platybasia, as mentioned earlier in this chapter. Robin sequence has been reported to occur in 17% of newborns with VCFS, and babies with VCFS make up 13% of all babies with Robin sequence (Shprintzen, 1988). Therefore, if a baby with

Robin sequence does not express another obvious multiple anomaly syndrome such as Stickler syndrome or Treacher Collins syndrome, FISH to rule out VCFS is indicated. The presence of congenital heart disease associated with Robin sequence would dramatically increase the probability that the baby has VCFS.

## DiGeorge Sequence

Like Robin sequence, the association of immune deficiency with thymic aplasia, hypocalcemia with hypoparathyroidism, and congenital heart disease is a developmental sequence instigated by a disruption in the development of the third and fourth pharyngeal pouches during embryogenesis. Labeled DiGeorge sequence in honor of Angelo DiGeorge, who discussed the condition in the literature as early as 1965, the condition was originally thought to be fatal in all cases because of the combination of severe immune deficiency and conotruncal heart anomalies (DiGeorge, 1965, 1968). Today, mortality in VCFS, even those cases with DiGeorge sequence, is uncommon. The combination of immune, endocrine, and cardiac anomalies has been recognized to be etiologically nonspecific and associated with a number of multiple anomaly syndromes including del 10p, del 17p, infants of diabetic mothers, Zellweger syndrome, peroxisomal disorders (Robin & Shprintzen, 2005), Down syndrome, Kabuki syndrome, fetal alcohol syndrome, CHARGE syndrome, and de Lange syndrome (Shprintzen, 2005b). Although many people refer to VCFS as DiGeorge syndrome, the reality is that DiGeorge is not a syndrome, but a sequence, and this particular sequence occurs less frequently in VCFS than Robin sequence. Fewer than 15% of individuals with VCFS meet the diagnostic criteria for DiGeorge (Shprintzen, 2005b). As mentioned previously, severe immune deficiency is uncommon in VCFS. Confounding the diagnostic label DiGeorge is the fact that the anomalies associated with this sequence can happen intermittently and will vary over time. Hypocalcemia and hypoparathyroidism may not be present at birth but can develop later in life, including adulthood. Hypocalcemia may similarly come and go with little evidence of problems in childhood, or conversely, hypocalcemia may resolve spontaneously and permanently in some infants.

## Potter Sequence

Potter sequence is a fatal grouping of anomalies triggered by bilateral renal agenesis, although some clinicians also include other causes of reduced fetal urinary output as factors, including urethral obstructions, polycystic kidneys, and other causes of oligohydramnios (reduced amniotic fluid). Potter sequence results in a variety of deformations caused by abnormal compression of the fetus because of the lack of an appropriate amniotic fluid environment for the fetus. Normal amounts of amniotic fluid are dependent on adequate urine output by the fetus, so renal agenesis will prevent the normal production and maintenance of the fluid environment for the fetus. The characteristic facial appearance of the newborn or fetus with Potter sequence includes a flattening of the nose, retrognathia, prominent epicanthal folds and redundant folds of skin under the eyes, and low-set, flattened ears. Pulmonary problems are also common. In severe cases there is sirenomelia (fusion of the legs). Most cases of Potter sequence result in stillbirths or death shortly after birth, although in rare cases with less severe renal anomalies, survival is possible.

## Holoprosencephaly

Holoprosencephaly is a developmental anomaly of the brain that results in incomplete or absent septation and separation of the hemispheres (Figure 2–72). In severe cases, the brain is a single sphere rather than two hemispheres, with no differentiation of ventricles (Figure 2–72). In milder cases, there is partial differentiation of the hemispheres. Olfactory tracts are often absent and the brain is typically abnormal in size and function. Diabetes insipidus often accompanies holoprosencephaly, as does pituitary hypoplasia or agenesis. Ocular malformations may also be associated with holoprosencephaly, even in its milder forms, including iris and optic nerve colobomas (see Figure 2–32). In severe cases of holoprosencephaly, the condition is incompatible with life. The first report of holoprosencephaly associated with VCFS was by Wraith et al. (1985), as discussed earlier in the section on brain malformations. Holoprosencephaly may be underdetected in VCFS because most babies with

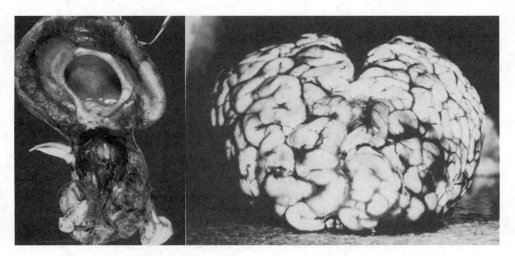

**FIGURE 2–72.** Brain with holoprosencephaly with no hemisphere differentiation (known as alobar holoprosencephaly, *left*) and a brain with incomplete septation of the frontal lobes (*right*), demonstrating partially lobar holoprosencephaly.

holoprosencephaly do not survive beyond the neonatal period, and FISH for a chromosome 22q11.2 deletion is not typically performed on these cases in the differential diagnosis.

## WHY THE EXPANSIVE PHENOTYPE?

The number of anomalies reported to be associated with VCFS here and in other publications is possibly the largest number of findings associated with any syndrome. There are several possible explanations for this. One is that the majority of individuals with VCFS have 40 genes missing on one copy of chromosome 22 and a smaller percentage have over 30 genes missing. This is a large number of genes that may alter the expression of the region within chromosome 22, and these genes may be important for human development and human performance. However, it should be kept in mind that there are many other syndromes that have genomic rearrangements that involve a similar number or even a larger number of genes. Some syndromes involve trisomies of entire chromosomes (such as Down syndrome), others the deletion of entire chromosomes (such as Turner syndrome), without as many anomalies catalogued for the disorder.

Another possibility is that so many anomalies have been reported because the syndrome has been the source of so much scrutiny. The instigation for this intense study was clearly the report of psychiatric illness associated with VCFS (Shprintzen et al., 1992), because this was the first hard genetic link to the development of psychosis, and it is recognized that VCFS remains the single most potent genetic factor for predicting mental illness. The large number of anomalies associated with VCFS may be the by-product of the large number of scientists who turned their attention to VCFS after 1992 as is evident from the thousands of publications about the syndrome in less than 15 years.

Another possibility is that many of the anomalies in VCFS represent developmental sequences and vascular disruption anomalies as reported by Shprintzen et al. (1997). Because fetal development is so heavily dependent on normal vascular supply, and because vascular anomalies are ubiquitous in VCFS, it is possible that many of the findings, such as the appearance of the ears, the fingertips, absence of the kidneys, brain anomalies, structural anomalies of the palate and pharynx, and more, are related to abnormalities of vascular supply.

Regardless of the reason for the large number of clinical findings in VCFS, the message is clear. Clinicians need to be able to address these problems with appropriate triage to other specialists, and preferably within the confines of an interdisciplinary team. Without comprehensive evaluation, comprehensive treatment is not possible.

## VIDEOS IN THIS CHAPTER

**Video 2–1:** Nasopharyngoscopy and videofluoroscopy of a child with VCFS and occult submucous cleft palate compared to a normal.

**Video 2–2:** Multi-view videofluoroscopy of a child with VCFS compared to a normal.

**Video 2–3:** Asymmetric velar structure and movement as seen both endoscopically and in videofluoroscopy.

**Video 2–4:** Asymmetry of the pharynx in VCFS on nasopharyngoscopic examination.

**Video 2–5:** Asymmetric movement of the lateral pharyngeal walls as seen in frontal view videofluoroscopy.

**Video 2–6:** Dilation of the Eustachian tube orifice during swallowing as the belly of the levator lifts the torus tubarius in a normal individual.

**Video 2–7:** Lack of dilation of the Eustachian tube orifice during swallowing in an individual with VCFS. Note that the torus is relatively immobile and the belly of the levator fills the orifice of the tube because it is positioned abnormally compared to the normal.

**Video 2–8:** Lateral view videofluoroscopy of a normal 5-year-old child showing the velum making contact with the adenoid pad, not the posterior pharyngeal wall, in order to achieve velopharyngeal closure compared to a lateral view videofluoroscopy of a 5-year-old child with VCFS showing a much smaller adenoid and failure for the velum to contact the adenoid pad even though the palate is mobile.

**Video 2–9:** Hypertrophic tonsils in VCFS. Note the contact between the tonsil and the epiglottis.

**Video 2–10:** Laryngomalacia in VCFS.

**Video 2–11:** Asymmetric arytenoid and corniculate cartilages in a 5-year-old with VCFS.

**Video 2–12:** Asymmetric pharynx showing increased fullness in the posterior pharyngeal wall on the right side.

**Video 2–13:** Vocal cord paresis and vocal cord paralysis in VCFS.

**Video 2–14:** Infant with VCFS and Robin sequence feeding. Note the chest retractions and effort expended during feeding.

**Video 2–15:** Asymmetric pharynx in VCFS resulting in compromise of the pyroform sinus on the side with increased fullness.

**Video 2–16:** Pulsation of the internal carotid artery in the hypopharynx making contact with the aryepiglottic fold.

**Video 2–17:** Videofluoroscopy and nasopharyngoscopy of a child with VCFS who has gross velopharyngeal insufficiency and glottal stop substitutions, followed by a study of a child with gross VPI and no glottal stop substitutions. The third segment show a child with VCFS with movement in the velopharyngeal valve and a relatively small gap, but perceptually severe hypernasality.

**Video 2–18:** A child with VCFS with ubiquitous glottal stop substitutions for all sounds except nasal consonants.

## REFERENCES

Al-Khattat, A. (2007). Leg pain: 3 year prospective study. Retrieved 12/2/07 from http://www.vcfsef.org/pp/3YearProspectiveStudy/index.htm

Altman, D. H., Altman, N. R., Mitnick, R. J., & Shprintzen, R. J. (1994). Further delineation of brain anomalies in velo-cardio-facial syndrome. *American Journal of Medical Genetics* (Neuropsychiatric Section), *54*, 174–175.

American Academy of Family Physicians. (2007). Retrieved 12/2/07 from http://www.aafp.org/afp/20030901/879.html

American Psychiatric Association. (1994). *Diagnostic and statistical manual of mental disorders* (4th ed.). Washington, DC: Author.

Anaclerio, S., Di Ciommo, V., Michielon, G., Digilio, M. C., Formigari, R., Picchio, F. M., et al. (2004). Conotruncal heart defects: Impact of genetic syndromes on immediate operative mortality. *Italian Heart Journal*, *5*, 624–628.

Aneja, A., Fremont, W. P., Antshel, K. M., Faraone, S. V., Abdul Sabur, N., Higgins, A. M., et al. (2007). Manic symptoms and behavioral dysregulation in youth with velocardiofacial syndrome (22q11.2 deletion syndrome). *Journal of Child and Adolescent Psychopharmacology*, *17*, 105–114.

Antshel, K. M., Abdul Sabur, N., Roizen, N., Fremont, W., & Kates, W. R. (2005). Sex differences in cognitive functioning in velocardiofacial syndrome (VCFS). *Developmental Neuropsychology*, *28*, 849–869.

Antshel, K. M., Aneja, A., Strunge, L., Peebles, J., Fremont, W. P., Stallone, K., et al. (2006). Autistic spectrum disorders in velo-cardio facial syndrome (22q11.2 deletion). *Journal of Autism and Developmental Disorders*, *37*, 1776–1786

Antshel, K., Fremont, W., Higgins, A. M., Shprintzen, R. J., & Kates, W. R. (2006). ADHD, major depressive disorder, and simple phobias are prevalent psychiatric conditions in youth with velocardiofacial syndrome (VCFS). *Journal of the American Academy of Child and Adolescent Psychiatry*, *45*, 596–603.

Antshel, K. M., Stallone, K., Abdul Sabur, N., Roizen, N., Higgins, A. M., Shprintzen, R. J., et al. (2007). Temperament in velocardiofacial syndrome. *Journal of Intellectual Disability Research*, *51*, 218–227.

Argamaso, R. V., Levandowski, G. J., Golding-Kushner, K. J., & Shprintzen, R. J. (1994). Treatment of asymmetric velopharyngeal insufficiency with skewed pharyngeal flap. *Cleft Palate—Craniofacial Journal*, *31*, 287–294.

Arnold, J. S., Braunstein, E. M., Ohyama, T., Groves, A. K., Adams, J. C., Brown, M. C., et al. (2006). Tissue-specific roles of Tbx1 in the development of the outer, middle and inner ear, defective in 22q11DS patients. *Human Molecular Genetics*, *15*, 1629–1639.

Arvystas, M., & Shprintzen, R.J. (1984). Craniofacial morphology in the velo-cardio-facial syndrome. *Journal of Craniofacial Genetics & Developmental Biology*, *4*, 39–45.

Bache, I., Nielsen, N. M., Rostgaard, K., Tommerup, N., & Frisch, M. (2007). Autoimmune diseases in a Danish cohort of 4,866 carriers of constitutional structural chromosomal rearrangements. *Arthritis & Rheumatism*, *56*, 2402–2409.

Baker, K. D., & Skuse, D. H. (2005). Adolescents and young adults with 22q11 deletion syndrome: Psychopathology in an at-risk group. *British Journal of Psychiatry*, *186*, 115–120.

Barnea-Goraly, N., Menon, V., Krasnow, B., Ko, A., Reiss, A., & Eliez S. (2003). Investigations of white matter structure in velocardiofacial syndrome: A diffusion tensor imaging study. *American Journal of Psychiatry*, 1863–1869.

Bassett, A. S., Chow, E. W. C., Abdel Malik, P., Gheorghiu, M., Husted, J., & Weksberg, R. (2003). The schizophrenia phenotype in 22q11 deletion syndrome. *American Journal of Psychiatry*, *160*, 1580–1586.

Bawle, E. V., Conard, J., Van Dyke, D. L., Czarnecki, P., & Driscoll, D. A. (1998). Seven new cases of Cayler cardiofacial syndrome with chromosome 22q11.2 deletion, including a familial case. *American Journal of Medical Genetics*, *79*, 406–410.

Bingham, P. M., Zimmerman, R. A., McDonald-McGinn, D., Driscoll, D., Emanuel, B. S., & Zackai, E. (1997). Enlarged Sylvian fissures in infants with interstitial deletion of chromosome 22q11. *American Journal of Medical Genetics*, *74*, 538–543.

Bird, L. M. (2001). Cortical dysgenesis and 22q11 deletion. *Clinical Dysmorphology*, *10*, 77.

Bird, L. M., & Scambler, P. (2000). Cortical dysgenesis in 2 patients with chromosome 22q11 deletion. *Clinical Genetics*, *58*, 64–68.

Bluestone, C. D. (1971). Eustachian tube obstruction in the infant with cleft palate. *Annals of Otology, Rhinology & Laryngology*, *80*(Suppl. 2), 1–30.

Budarf, M. L., Konkle, B. A., Ludlow, L. B., Michaud, D., Yamashiro, D. J., McDonald McGinn, D., et al. (1995). Identification of a patient with Bernard-Soulier syndrome and a deletion in the DiGeorge/velo-cardio-facial chromosomal region in 22q11.2. *Human Molecular Genetics*, *4*, 763–766.

Camp, B. W., Broman, S. H., Nichols, P. L., & Leff, M. (1998). Maternal and neonatal risk factors for mental retardation: Defining the "at-risk" child. *Early Human Development*, *50*, 159–173.

Cayler, G. G. (1969). Cardiofacial syndrome. *Archives of Disease in Childhood*, *44*, 69–75.

Center for Disease Control and Prevention (2007). Retrieved from http://www.cdc.gov/ncbddd/autism/addm.htm

Chegar, B. E., Shprintzen, R. J., Curtis, M. S., & Tatum, S. A. (2007). Pharyngeal flap and obstructive apnea: Maximizing speech outcome while limiting complications. *Archives of Facial and Plastic Surgery*, *9*, 252–259.

Chegar, B. E., Tatum, S. A., Marrinan, E., & Shprintzen, R. J. (2006). Upper airway asymmetry in velo-cardio-facial syndrome. *International Journal of Pediatric Otorhinolaryngology*, *70*, 1375–1381.

Choi, J. H., Shin, Y. L., Kim, G. H., Seo, E. J., Kim, Y., Park, I. S., et al. (2005). Endocrine manifestations of chromosome 22q11.2 microdeletion syndrome. *Hormone Research, 63,* 294–299.

Chow, E. W., Mikulis, D. J., Zipursky, R. B., Scutt, L, E., Weksberg, R., & Bassett, A. S. (1999). Qualitative MRI findings in adults with 22q11 deletion syndrome and schizophrenia. *Biological Psychiatry, 46,* 1436–1442.

Chow, E. W., Zipursky, R. B., Mikulis, D. J., & Bassett, A. S. (2002). Structural brain abnormalities in patients with schizophrenia and 22q11 deletion syndrome. *Biological Psychiatry, 51,* 208–215.

Chu, W. C. W., & Metreweli, C. (2002). Ectopic thymic tissue in the paediatric age group. *Acta Radiologica, 43,* 144–146.

Cohen, M. M., Jr. (1999). Robin sequences and complexes: Causal heterogeneity and pathogenetic/phenotypic variability. *American Journal of Medical Genetics, 84,* 311–315.

Cook, E. H., Stein, M. A., Krasowski, M. D., Cox, N. J., Olken, D. M., Kieffer, J. E., et al. (1995). Association of attention deficit disorder and the dopamine transporter gene. *American Journal of Human Genetics, 56,* 993–998.

Debbane, M., Schaer, M., Farhoumand, R., Glaser, B., & Eliez, S. (2006). Hippocampal volume reduction in 22q11.2 deletion syndrome. *Neuropsychologia, 44,* 2360–2365.

Devriendt, K., Thienen, M. N., Swillen, A., & Fryns, J. P. (1996). Cerebellar hypoplasia in a patient with velo-cardio-facial syndrome. *Developmental Medicine and Child Neurology, 38,* 949–953.

Dickson, D. R. (1976). Anatomy of the normal and cleft palate Eustachian tube. *Annals of Otology, Rhinology & Laryngology, 85*(2 Suppl. 25, Pt. 2), 25–29.

Diehl, D. J., & Gershon, S. (1992). The role of dopamine in mood disorders. *Comprehensive Psychiatry, 33,* 115–120.

DiGeorge, A. M. (1965). A new concept of the cellular basis of immunity. *Journal of Pediatrics, 67,* 907.

DiGeorge, A. M. (1968). Congenital absence of the thymus and its immunologic consequences: Concurrence with congenital hypoparathyroidism. *Birth Defects Original Article Series, 4*(1), 116–121.

Ehara, H., Maegaki, Y., & Takeshita, K. (2003). Pachygyria and polymicrogyria in 22q11 deletion syndrome. *American Journal of Medical Genetics, 117,* 80–82.

Eicher, P. S., McDonald-McGinn, D. M., Fox, C. A., Driscoll, D. A., Emanuel, B. S., & Zackai, E. H. (2000). Dysphagia in children with a 22q11.2 deletion: Unusual pattern found on modified barium swallow. *Journal of Pediatrics, 137,* 158–164.

Eliez, S. (2007). Autism in children with 22q11.2 deletion syndrome. *Journal of the American Academy of Child and Adolescent Psychiatry, 46,* 433–434.

Eliez, S., Schmitt, J. E., White, C. D., & Reiss, A. L. (2000). Children and adolescents with velocardiofacial syndrome: A volumetric MRI study. *American Journal of Psychiatry, 157,* 409–415.

Eliez, S., Schmitt, J. E., White, C. D., Wellis, V. G., & Reiss, A. L. (2001). A quantitative MRI study of posterior fossa development in velocardiofacial syndrome. *Biological Psychiatry, 49,* 540–546.

Feinstein, C., Eliez, S., Blasey, C., & Reiss, A. L. (2002). Psychiatric disorders and behavioral problems in children with velocardiofacial syndrome: Usefulness as phenotypic indicators of schizophrenia risk. *Biological Psychiatry, 51,* 312–318.

Fitch, N. (1983). Velo-cardio-facial syndrome and eye abnormality. *American Journal of Medical Genetics, 15,* 669.

Galarza, M., Merlo, A. B., Ingratta, A., Albanese, E. F., & Albanese, A. M. (2004). Cavum septum pellucidum and its increased prevalence in schizophrenia: A neuroembryological classification. *Journal of Neuropsychiatry and Clinical Neuroscience, 16*, 41–46.

Gereau, S. A., & Shprintzen, R. J. (1988). The role of adenoids in the development of normal speech following palate repair. *Laryngoscope, 98*, 299–303.

Gereau, S. A., Steven, D., Bassila, M., Sher, A. E., Sidoti, E. J., Jr., Morgan, M., et al. (1988). Endoscopic observations of Eustachian tube abnormalities in children with palatal clefts. In D. J. Lim, C. D. Bluestone, J. O. Klein, & J. D. Nelson (Eds.), *Symposium on otitis media* (pp. 60–63). Toronto: B. C. Decker.

Goldberg, R., Motzkin, B., Marion, R., Scambler, P. J., & Shprintzen, R. J. (1993). Velo-cardio-facial syndrome: A review of 120 patients. *American Journal of Medical Genetics, 45*, 313–319.

Golding-Kushner, K. J. (1991). *Craniofacial morphology and velopharyngeal physiology in four syndromes of clefting.* Unpublished doctoral dissertation, The Graduate School and University Center, City University of New York.

Golding-Kushner, K. J. (2000). *Therapy techniques for cleft palate speech and related disorders.* San Diego, CA: Singular.

Golding-Kushner, K. J. (2005). Speech and language disorders in velo-cardio-facial syndrome. In K. Murphy & P. Scambler (Eds.), *Velo-cardio-facial syndrome: A model for understanding microdeletion disorders* (pp. 181–199). Cambridge, UK: Cambridge University Press.

Golding-Kushner, K. J., Argamaso, R. V., Cotton, R. T., Grames, L. M., Henningsson, G., Jones, D. L., et al. (1990). Standardization for the reporting of nasopharyngoscopy and multi-view videofluoroscopy: A report from an international working group. *Cleft Palate Journal, 27*, 337–347.

Golding-Kushner, K., Weller, G., & Shprintzen, R. J. (1985). Velo-cardio-facial syndrome: Language and psychological profiles. *Journal of Craniofacial Genetics and Developmental Biology, 5*, 259–266.

Goldmuntz, E., Clark, B. J., Mitchell, L. E., Jawad, A. F., Cuneo, B. F., Reed, L., et al. (1998). Frequency of 22q11 deletions in patients with conotruncal defects. *Journal of the American College of Cardiology, 32*, 492–498.

Gosselin, J., Lebon-Labich, B., Lucron, H., Marçon, F., & Leheup, B. (2004). Syndrome de délétion 22q11 et maladie de Basedow. À propos de trois observations pédiatriques. *Archives Pédiatriques, 11*, 1468–1471.

Gothelf, D., Feinstein, C., Thompson, T., Gu, E., Penniman, L., Van Stone, E., et al. (2007). Risk factors for the emergence of psychotic disorders in adolescents with 22q11.2 deletion syndrome. *American Journal of Psychiatry, 164*, 663–669.

Gothelf, D., Presburger, G., Levy, D., Nahmani, A., Burg, M., Berant, M., et al. (2004). Genetic, developmental, and physical factors associated with attention deficit hyperactivity disorder in patients with velocardiofacial syndrome. *American Journal of Medical Genetics, Part B: Neuropsychiatric Genetics, 126*, 116–121.

Graf, W. D., Unis, A. S., Yates, C. M., Sulzbacher, S., Dinulos, M. B., Jack, R. M., et al. (2001). Catecholamines in patients with 22q11.2 deletion syndrome and the low-activity *COMT* polymorphism. *Neurology, 57*, 410–416.

Havkin, N., Tatum, S. A., III, & Shprintzen, R. J. (2000). Velopharyngeal insufficiency and articulation impairment in velo-cardio-facial syndrome: The influence of adenoids on phonemic development. *International Journal of Pediatric Otorhinolaryngology, 54*, 103–110.

Henningsson, G., & Isberg, A. (1991). A cineradiographic study of velopharyngeal movements for deviant versus nondeviant articulation. *Cleft Palate-Craniofacial Journal, 28*, 115–117.

Heyman, S., Eicher, P. S., & Alavi, A. (1995). Radionuclide studies of the upper gastrointestinal tract in children with feeding disorders. *Journal of Nuclear Medicine, 36*, 351–354.

Horowitz, A., Shifman, S., Rivlin, N., Pisanté, A., & Darvasi, A. (2005). A survey of the 22q11 microdeletion in a large cohort of schizophrenia patients. *Schizophrenia Research, 73*, 263–267.

Kahn, R. S., & Davis, K. L. (1995). New developments in dopamine and schizophrenia. In F. Bloom & D. Kupfer (Eds.), *Psychopharmacology: The fourth generation of progress* (pp. 1193–1203). New York: Raven Press Ltd.

Kanner, L. (1943). Autistic disturbances of affective contact. *The Nervous Child, 2*, 217–250.

Kao, A., Mariani, J., McDonald-McGinn, D.M. , Maisenbacher, M.K., Brooks-Kayal A.R., Zackai, E.H. et al. (2004). Increased prevalence of unprovoked seizures in patients with a 22q11.2 deletion. *American Journal of Medical Genetics, 129A*, 29–34.

Kaplan, E. N. (1975). The occult submucous cleft palate. *Cleft Palate Journal, 12*(4), 356–368.

Karayiorgou, M., Morris, M. A., Morrow, B., Shprintzen, R. J., Goldberg, R., Borrow, J., et al. (1995). Schizophrenia susceptibility associated with interstitial deletions of chromosome 22q11. *Proceedings of the National Academy of Science, 92*, 7612–7616.

Kates, W. R., Antshel, K., Roizen, N., Fremont, W., & Shprintzen, R. J. (2005). Velo-cardio-facial syndrome. In M. G. Butler & F. J. Meaney (Eds.), *Genetics of developmental disabilities* (pp 383–418.). New York: Marcel Dekker.

Kates, W. R., Antshel, K., Willhite, R., Bessette, B. A., Abdul Sabur, N., & Higgins, A. M. (2005). Gender moderated dorsolateral prefrontal reductions in 22q11.2 deletion syndrome: Implications for risk for schizophrenia. *Neuropsychology and Developmental Cognition, Part C: Child Neuropsychology, 11*, 73–85.

Kates, W. R., Burnette, C. P., Bessette, B. A., Folley, B. S., Strunge, L., Jabs, E. W., et al. (2004). Frontal and caudate alterations in velocardiofacial syndrome (deletion at chromosome 22q11.2). *Journal of Child Neurology, 19*, 337–342.

Kates, W. R., Miller, A. M., Abdul Sabur, N., Antshel, K. M., Conchelos, J., Fremont, W., et al. (2006). Temporal lobe anatomy and psychiatric symptoms in velocardiofacial syndrome (22q11.2 deletion syndrome). *Journal of the American Academy of Child and Adolescent Psychiatry, 45*, 587–595.

Kawame, H., Adachi, M., Tachibana, K., Kurosawa, K., Ito, F., Gleason, M. M., et al. (2001). Graves' disease in patients with 22q11.2 deletion. *Journal of Pediatrics, 139*, 892–895.

Kerstjens-Frederikse, W. S., Hofstra, R. M. W., van Essen, A. J., Meijers, J. H. C., Buys, C. H. C. M. (1999). A Hirschsprung disease locus at 22q11? *Journal of Medical Genetics, 36*, 221–224.

Klingberg, G., Dietz, W., Oskarsdottir, S., Odelius, H., Gelander, L., & Noren, J. G. (2005). Morphological appearance and chemical composition of enamel in primary teeth from patients with 22q11 deletion syndrome. *European Journal of Oral Science, 113*, 303–311.

Klingberg, G., Oskarsdottir, S., Johannesson, E. L., & Noren, J. G. (2002). Oral manifestations in 22q11 deletion syndrome. *International Journal of Paediatric Dentistry, 12*, 14–23.

Koolen, D. A., Veltman, J. A., Renier, W. O., Droog, R. P., van Kessel, A. G., & de Vries, B. B. A. (2004). Chromosome 22q11 deletion and pachygyria characterized by array-based comparative genomic hybridization. *American Journal of Medical Genetics, 131A*, 322–324.

Krahn, L. E., Maraganore, D. M., & Michels, V. V. (1998). Childhood onset schizophrenia associated with parkinsonism in a patient with a microdeletion of chromosome 22. *Mayo Clinic Proceedings, 73*, 956–959.

Lachman, H. M., Morrow, B., Shprintzen, R. J., Veit, S., Parsia, S. S., Faedda, G., et al. (1996). Association of codon 108/158 catechol-o-methyl transferase gene polymorphism with the psychiatric manifestations of VCFS. *American Journal of Medical Genetics, 67*, 468–472.

Lipson, A. H., Yuille, D., Angel, M., Thompson, P. G., Vanderwoord, J. G., & Beckenham, E. J. (1991). Velo-cardio-facial syndrome: An important syndrome for the dysmorphologist to recognize. *Journal of Medical Genetics, 28*, 596–604.

Ludlow, L. B., Schick, B. P., Budarf, M. L., Driscoll, D. A., Zackai, E. H., Cohen, A., et al. (1996). Identification of a mutation in a GATA binding site of the platelet glycoprotein Ibb promoter resulting in the Bernard-Soulier syndrome. *Journal of Biological Chemistry, 271*, 22076–22080.

Lynch, D. R., McDonald-McGinn, D. M., Zackai, E. H., Emanuel, B. S., Driscoll, D. A., Whitaker, L. A., et al. (1996). Cerebellar atrophy in a patient with velocardiofacial syndrome. *Journal of Medical Genetics, 33*, 719–720.

MacKenzie-Stepner, K., Witzel, M. A., Stringer, D. A., Lindsay, W. K., Munro, I. R., & Hughes, H. (1987). Abnormal carotid arteries in the velocardiofacial syndrome: A report of three cases. *Plastic and Reconstructive Surgery, 80*, 347–351.

Mansour, A., Wang, F., Goldberg, R., & Shprintzen, R. J. (1987). Ocular findings in the velo-cardio-facial syndrome. *Journal of Pediatric Ophthalmology, 24*, 263–266.

McElhinney, D. B., Driscoll, D. A., Levin, E. R., Jawad, A. F., Emanuel, B. S., & Goldmuntz, E. (2003). Chromosome 22q11 deletion in patients with ventricular septal defect: Frequency and associated cardiovascular anomalies. *Pediatrics, 112*, e472–e476.

Medline Plus. (2007). Retrieved 12/2/07 from http://www.nlm.nih.gov/medlineplus/ency/article/000991.htm

Ming, J. E., McDonald-McGinn, D. M., Megerian, T. E., Driscoll, D. A., Elias, E. R., Russell, B. R., et al. (1997). Skeletal anomalies and deformities in patients with deletions of 22q11. *American Journal of Medical Genetics 72*, 210–215.

Mitnick, R. J., Bello, J. A., Golding-Kushner, K. J., Argamaso, R. V., & Shprintzen, R. J. (1996). The use of magnetic resonance angiography prior to pharyngeal flap surgery in patients with velo-cardio-facial syndrome. *Plastic and Reconstructive Surgery, 97*, 908–919.

Mitnick, R. J., Bello, J. A., & Shprintzen, R. J. (1994). Brain anomalies in velo-cardio-facial syndrome. *American Journal of Medical Genetics (Neuropsychiatric Section), 54*, 100–106.

Miyamoto, R. C., Cotton, R. T., Rope, A. F., Hopkin, R. J., Cohen, A. P., Shott, S. R., et al. (2004). Association of anterior glottic webs with velocardiofacial syndrome (chromosome 22q11.2 deletion). *Otolaryngology–Head & Neck Surgery, 130*, 415–417.

Moss, E., Batshaw, M., Solot, C., Gerdes, M., McDonald-McGinn, D., Driscoll, D., et al. (1999). Psychoeducational profile of the 22q11.2 microdeletion: A complex pattern. *Journal of Pediatrics, 134,* 193–198.

Moss, M. L. (1975). New studies of cranial growth. *Birth Defects, 11,* 283–295.

Moss, M. L., & Rankow, R. M. (1968). The role of the functional matrix in mandibular growth. *Angle Orthodontist, 38,* 95–103.

Motzkin, B., Marion, R., Goldberg, R., Shprintzen, R. J., & Saenger, P. (1993). Variable phenotypes in velocardiofacial syndrome with chromosomal deletion. *Journal of Pediatrics, 123,* 406–410.

Murphy, K. C., Jones, L. A., & Owen, M. J. (1999). High rates of schizophrenia in adults with velo-cardio-facial syndrome. *Archives of General Psychiatry, 56,* 940–945.

Nemours Foundation, Kids Health for Parents. (2007). Retrieved 12/2/07 from http://www.kidshealth.org/parent/nutrition_fit/nutrition/failure_thrive.html

Nickel, R. E., & Magenis, R. E. (1996). Neural tube defects and deletions of 22q11. *American Journal of Medical Genetics, 66,* 25–27.

O'Hanlon, J. F., Ritchie, R. C., Smith, E. A., & Patel, R. (2003). Replacement of antipsychotic and antiepileptic medication by L-alpha-methyldopa in a woman with velocardiofacial syndrome. *International Clinical Psychopharmacology, 18,* 117–119.

Papolos, D. F., Faedda, G. L., Veit, S., Goldberg, R., Morrow, B., Kucherlapati, R., et al. (1996). Bipolar spectrum disorders in patients diagnosed with velo-cardio-facial syndrome: Does a hemizygous deletion of chromosome 22q11 result in bipolar affective disorder? *American Journal of Psychiatry, 153,* 1541–1547.

Pettersson, A., Richiardi, L., Nordenskjold, A., Kaijser, M., & Akre, O. (2007). Age at surgery for undescended testis and risk of testicular cancer. *New England Journal of Medicine, 356,* 1835–1841.

Pulver, A. E., Nestadt, G., Goldberg, R., Shprintzen, R. J., Lamacz, M., Wolyniec, P. S., et al. (1994). Psychotic illness in patients diagnosed with velo-cardio-facial syndrome and their relatives. *Journal of Nervous and Mental Disorders, 182,* 476–478.

Rasmussen, S. A., Williams, C. A., Ayoub, E. M., Sleasman, J. W., Gray, B. A., Bent-Williams, A., et al. (1996). Juvenile rheumatoid arthritis in velo-cardio-facial syndrome: Coincidence or unusual complication? *American Journal of Medical Genetics, 64,* 546–550.

Reyes, M. R. T., LeBlanc, E. M., & Bassila, M. K. (1999). Hearing loss and otitis media in velo-cardio-facial syndrome. *International Journal of Pediatric Otorhinolaryngology, 47,* 227–233.

Ricchetti, E. T., States, L., Hosalkar, H. S., Tamai, J., Maisenbacher, M., McDonald-McGinn, D. M., et al. (2004). SyndromeRadiographic study of the upper cervical spine in the 22q11.2 deletion. *Journal of Bone and Joint Surgery (American), 86,* 1751–1760.

Robin, N. H., & Shprintzen, R. J. (2005). Defining the clinical spectrum of deletion 22q11.2. *Journal of Pediatrics, 147,* 90–96.

Robin, N. H., Taylor, C. J., McDonald-McGinn, D. M., Zackai, E. H., Bingham, P., Collins, K. J, et al. (2006). Polymicrogyria and deletion 22q11.2 syndrome: Window to the etiology of a common cortical malformation. *American Journal of Medical Genetics, Part A, 140,* 2416–2425.

Rommel, N., Vantrappen, G., Swillen, A., Devriendt, K., Feenstra, L., & Fryns, J. P. (1999). Retrospective analysis of feeding and speech disorders in 50 patients with velo-cardio-facial syndrome. *Genetic Counseling, 10,* 71–78.

Ryan, A. K., Goodship, J. A., Wilson, D. I., Philip, N., Levy, A., Seidel, H., et al. (1997). Spectrum of clinical features associated with interstitial chromosome 22q11 deletions: A European collaborative study. *Journal of Medical Genetics, 34*, 798–804.

Salyer, K. E., Song, K. W., & Sperry, E. E. (2006). Two-flap palatoplasty: 20-year experience and evolution of surgical technique. *Plastic and Reconstructive Surgery, 118*, 193–204.

Scambler, P. J., Kelly, D., Lindsay, E., Williamson, R., Goldberg, R., Shprintzen, R. J., et al. (1992). Velo-cardio-facial syndrome associated with chromosome 22 deletions encompassing the DiGeorge locus. *Lancet, 339*, 1138–1139.

Scherer, N., D'Antonio, L., & Kalbfleisch, J. (1999). Early speech and language development in children with velocardiofacial syndrome. *American Journal of Medical Genetics, 88*, 714–723.

Sedláčková, E. (1955). Insufficiency of palatolaryngeal passage as a developmental disorder. *Časopis lékařů českých, 94*(12), 1304–1307.

Shashi, V., Muddasani, S., Santos, C. C., Berry, M. N., Kwapil, T. R., Lewandowski, E., et al. (2004). Abnormalities of the corpus callosum in nonpsychotic children with chromosome 22q11 deletion syndrome. *Neuroimage, 21*, 1399–1406.

Shprintzen, R. J. (1982). Palatal and pharyngeal anomalies in craniofacial syndromes. *Birth Defects, 18*(1), 53–78.

Shprintzen, R. J. (1988). Pierre Robin, micrognathia, and airway obstruction: The dependency of treatment on accurate diagnosis. *International Anesthesiology Clinic, 26*, 64–71.

Shprintzen, R. J. (1999). The Velo-Cardio-Facial Syndrome Educational Foundation Clinical Database Project. Retrieved 12/2/07 from http://www.vcfsef.org/pp/vcf_facts/index.htm

Shprintzen, R. J. (2000a). Velocardiofacial syndrome. *Otolaryngology Clinics of North America, 33*, 1217–1240.

Shprintzen, R. J. (2000b). Velo-cardio-facial syndrome: A distinctive behavioral phenotype. *Mental Retardation and Developmental Disabilities Research Reviews, 6*, 142–147.

Shprintzen, R. J. (2005). Velo-cardio-facial syndrome. *Progress in Pediatric Cardiology, 20*, 187–193.

Shprintzen, R. (2005). Velo-cardio-facial syndrome. In S. Cassidy & J. Allanson (Eds.), *Management of genetic syndromes* (pp. 615–632). New York: John Wiley & Sons.

Shprintzen, R. J., & Croft, C. B. (1981). Abnormalities of the Eustachian tube orifice in individuals with cleft palate. *International Journal of Pediatric Otorhinolaryngology, 3*, 15–23.

Shprintzen, R. J., Goldberg, R., Golding-Kushner, K. J., & Marion, R. (1992). Late-onset psychosis in the velo-cardio-facial syndrome. *American Journal of Medical Genetics, 42*, 141–142.

Shprintzen, R. J., Goldberg, R. B., Lewin, M. L., Sidoti, E. J., Berkman, M. D., Argamaso, R. V., et al. (1978). A new syndrome involving cleft palate, cardiac anomalies, typical facies, and learning disabilities: Velo-cardio-facial syndrome. *Cleft Palate Journal, 15*, 56–62.

Shprintzen, R. J., Goldberg, R., Young, D., & Wolford, L. (1981). The velo-cardio-facial syndrome: A clinical and genetic analysis. *Pediatrics, 67*, 167–172.

Shprintzen, R. J., Lewin, M. L., Croft, C. B., Daniller, A. I., Argamaso, R. V., Ship, A., et al. (1979). A comprehensive study of pharyngeal flap surgery: Tailor-made flaps. *Cleft Palate Journal, 16*, 46–55.

Shprintzen, R. J., Morrow, B., & Kucherlapati, R. (1997). Vascular anomalies may explain many of the features of velo-cardio-facial syndrome. *American Journal of Human Genetics, 61,* 34A.

Shprintzen, R. J., Schwartz, R., Daniller, A., & Hoch, L. (1985). The morphologic significance of bifid uvula. *Pediatrics, 75,* 553–561.

Shprintzen, R. J., Sher, A. E., & Croft, C. B. (1987). Hypernasal speech caused by hypertrophic tonsils. *International Journal of Pediatric Otorhinolaryngology, 14,* 45–56.

Shprintzen, R. J., & Singer, L. (1992). Upper airway obstruction and the Robin sequence. *International Anesthesiology Clinic, 30,* 109–114.

Shprintzen, R. J., Singer, L., Sidoti, E. J., & Argamaso, R. V. (1992). Pharyngeal flap surgery: Postoperative complications. *International Anesthesiology Clinic, 30,* 115–124.

Sidoti, E. J., & Shprintzen, R. J. (1995). Pediatric care and feeding of the newborn with a cleft. In R. J. Shprintzen & J. Bardach (Eds.), *Cleft palate speech management: A multidisciplinary approach* (pp. 63–74). St. Louis, MO: Mosby.

Skolnick, M. L., & McCall, G. N. (1972). Velopharyngeal competence and incompetence following pharyngeal flap surgery: A videofluoroscopic study in multiple projections. *Cleft Palate Journal, 9,* 1–12.

Sullivan, K. E., McDonald-McGinn, D. M., Driscoll, D. A., Zmijewski, C. M., Ellabban, A.S., Reed, L., et al. (1997). Juvenile rheumatoid arthritis-like polyarthritis in chromosome 22q11.2 deletion syndrome (DiGeorge anomalad/velocardiofacial syndrome/conotruncal anomaly face syndrome). *Arthritis & Rheumatism, 40,* 430–436.

Swillen, A., Devriendt, K., Legius, E., Eyskens, B., Dumoulin, M., Gewillig, M., et al. (1997). Intelligence and psychosocial adjustment in velocardiofacial syndrome: A study of 37 children and adolescents with VCFS. *Journal of Medical Genetics, 34,* 453–458.

Tatum, S. A., III, Chang, J., Havkin, N., & Shprintzen, R. J. (2002). Pharyngeal flap and the internal carotid in velo-cardio-facial syndrome. *Archives of Facial and Plastic Surgery, 4,* 73–80.

Usiskin, S. I., Nicolson, R., Krasnewich, D. M., Yan, W., Lenane, M., Wudarsky, M., et al. (1999). Velocardiofacial syndrome in childhood-onset schizophrenia. *Journal of the American Academy of Child and Adolescent Psychiatry, 38,* 1536–1543.

van Amelsvoort, T., Murphy, K. C., & Murphy, D. G. (2001). Chromosome 22q11 deletion and brain tissue composition. *British Journal of Psychiatry, 179,* 559.

Vargervik, K., Miller, A. J., Chierici, G., Harvold, E., & Tomer, B. S. (1984). Morphologic response to changes in neuromuscular patterns experimentally induced by altered modes of respiration. *American Journal of Orthodontics, 85,* 115–124.

Venail, F., Roux, A. F., Pallares-Ruiz, N., Claustres, M., Blanchet, P., Gardiner, Q., et al. (2004). Nonsyndromic 35 delG mutation of the connexin 26 gene associated with deafness in syndromic children: Two case reports. *Laryngoscope, 114,* 566–569.

Verhoeven, W. M., Tuinier, S., & Curfs, L. M. (2000). Prader-Willi psychiatric syndrome and velo-cardio-facial psychiatric syndrome. *Genetic Counseling, 11,* 205–213.

Verloes, A., Curry, C., Jamar, M., Herens, C., O'Lague, P., Marks, J., et al. (1998). Juvenile rheumatoid arthritis and del(22q11) syndrome: Non-random association. *Journal of Medical Genetics, 35,* 943–947.

Vorstman, J. A., Morcus, M. E., Duijff, S. N., Klaassen, P. W., Heineman-de Boer, J. A., Beemer, F. A., et al. (2006). The 22q11.2 deletion in children: High rate of autistic disorders and early onset of psychotic symptoms. *Journal of the American Academy of Child and Adolescent Psychiatry, 45,* 1104–1113.

Williams, M. A., Shprintzen, R. J., & Goldberg, R. B. (1985). Male-to-male transmission of the velo-cardio-facial syndrome: A case report and review of 60 cases. *Journal of Craniofacial and Genetic Development Biology, 5,* 175–180.

Williams, M. L., Shprintzen, R. J., & Rakoff, S. J. (1987). Adenoid hypoplasia in the velo-cardio-facial syndrome. *Journal of Craniofacial Genetics & Developmental Biology, 7,* 23–26.

Wolff, S. (2004). The history of autism. *European Child and Adolescent Psychiatry, 13,* 201–208.

Woodside, D. G., Linder-Aronson, S., Lundstrom, A., & McWilliam, J. (1991). Mandibular and maxillary growth after changed mode of breathing. *American Journal of Orthodontics and Dentofacial Orthopedics, 100,* 1–18.

Wraith, J. E., Super, M., Watson, G. H., & Phillips, M. (1985). Velo-cardio-facial syndrome presenting as holoprosencephaly. *Clinical Genetics, 27,* 408–410.

Young, D., Shprintzen, R. J., & Goldberg, R. (1980). Cardiac malformations in the velo-cardio-facial syndrome. *American Journal of Cardiology, 46,* 43–48.

Zim, S., Schelper, R., Kellman, R., Tatum, S., Ploutz-Snyder, R., & Shprintzen, R. J. (2003). Thickness and histologic and histochemical properties of the superior pharyngeal constrictor muscle in velocardiofacial syndrome. *Archives of Facial and Plastic Surgery, 5,* 503–507.

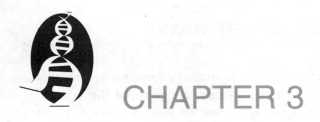

# CHAPTER 3

# The Genetics of VCFS

$W$hen 12 cases were first reported in 1978 (Shprintzen et al., 1978), VCFS was hypothesized to be an autosomal dominant genetic disorder because there was one instance of a mother to daughter transmission of the syndrome. Four more maternal transmissions of the syndrome were reported in 1981 (Shprintzen, Goldberg, Young, & Wolford, 1981), and then a father to son transmission in 1985 (Williams, Shprintzen, & Goldberg, 1985) ruled out X-linked transmission and confirmed that the syndrome was inherited as an autosomal dominant condition. At the time the pattern of inheritance was confirmed, microdeletions were just becoming known as causes of multiple anomaly syndromes, and only a few had been identified beginning in the mid-1980s. The initial hypothesis was that VCFS was a mutation of a single gene resulting in an autosomal dominant disorder.

As described in Chapter 1, Scambler et al. (1992) first reported that a deletion of DNA from chromosome 22 at the q11.2 band caused VCFS (see Figure 1–1), moving it into the category of a microdeletion syndrome, a type of disorder not even known in 1978. It was initially found that the deletion was large enough to contain multiple genes, but the specific details of the size of the deletion and the number and type of genes would unfold over subsequent years, as well as additional reports characterizing the deletion and the analysis of its genome. In 1992, our report of mental illness in VCFS that followed the discovery of the deletion provided additional impetus to pursue the deleted region because scientists were very interested in finding hard genetic causes for schizophrenia and other mental illnesses. Although mental illness may have been the impetus for the research, the large number of common anomalies associated with VCFS provided the potential for unraveling some of the causes for problems affecting large segments of the general population.

## WHAT DOES *GENETIC* MEAN?

Some people confuse the terms *genetic* and *hereditary* (or inherited). Genetic disorders refer to those that are caused by rearrangements of the DNA that result in anomalies. Those rearrangements could be deletions of DNA, extra DNA, alteration of the genetic code, or errors in the transcription or translation of the genetic code. Genetic disorders are not necessarily inherited. DNA often rearranges spontaneously, and in fact, this is most often the case in VCFS. More than 90% of new VCFS cases represent deletions that were not inherited from parents, representing de novo mutations (brand new rearrangements) in that individual. However, the syndrome in that child is still related back to the genome. That person who is affected may then have an affected child of his or her own in adult life. In this case, the disorder is both genetic and inherited.

### Mode of Inheritance

VCFS is inherited as an autosomal dominant disorder. Autosomal dominant means that the disorder is expressed with only one chromosome of the chromosome pair deleted. In other words, although there is one copy of a normal chromosome 22, the presence of the deletion on the other copy is sufficient to express the syndrome. When reproductive cells are formed, the process of meiotic cell division results in cells (eggs and sperm) that have single copies of each chromosome rather than pairs of each chromosome (Figure 3–1). Half of all of the reproductive cells that will be involved in passing on the parent's genome will therefore have a deleted copy of chromosome 22. Therefore, the probability of each pregnancy involving a person with VCFS is 50% because half of the reproductive cells have the deletion. In other words, for each pregnancy established, the chance that the fertilized egg and resulting child will have VCFS is the same as flipping a coin.

## DESCRIBING THE GENOME AT 22q11.2

The first challenge for researchers was to fully define the genome at 22q11.2 and determine where the breakpoints at both ends of the deletion were located. Researchers from a number of institutions competed and combined to accomplish this task, beginning in 1992. Study of the genome in this region continues to this day. The phases of that research were as follows:

1. To determine if all people with VCFS have the same deletion and how the deletion occurs.

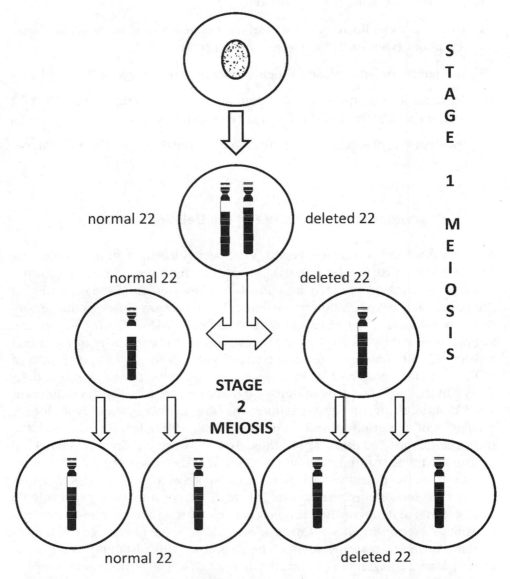

normal 22

deleted 22

normal 22

deleted 22

**STAGE
2
MEIOSIS**

normal 22

deleted 22

**FIGURE 3–1.** First stage of meiosis when cells go from diploid state (46 chromosomes in 23 pairs) to a haploid state (23 chromosomes in single copy). When
these cells become eggs and sperm, one half of them will have a deleted copy of
chromosome 22 that would result in a child with VCFS. In this figure the two copies
of chromosome 22 are shown, one deleted and one normal copy. Of the resulting
reproductive cells (sperm or eggs), half have a deleted copy of chromosome 22.

2. To identify all of the genes in the deleted region.

3. To determine what those genes do.

4. To identify candidate genes within the deleted region to determine how the phenotypes of the syndrome are expressed.

5. To identify polymorphisms (allelic variations) in the genes in 22q11.2.

6. To determine if there are any genetic effects outside of the 22q11.2 region that contribute to the phenotypic expressions.

7. To identify epigenetic factors that might contribute to the phenotypic spectrum.

### Determining the Nature of the Deletion in VCFS

As larger numbers of individuals with VCFS were identified, hundreds of DNA samples were analyzed by researchers to determine the consistency of the deletion size for all affected individuals. Morrow et al. (1995) found that the proximal breakpoint on chromosome 22 (the region closer to the centromere) was identical for nearly all individuals with VCFS (Figure 3–2). In the sample analyzed by Morrow et al., they found that the majority of cases had a deletion that spanned three million base pairs (3 megabases, or 3 Mb) of DNA. A smaller sample of VCFS cases, approximately 10% or less, had deletions half that size. It is now understood that there are actually three different sized deletions and that the deletions are caused by a unique evolutionary arrangement of chromosome 22 (Edelmann et al., 1999). It was also found that the large majority of cases, approximately 90%, were children of unaffected parents, meaning that the deletion was present in the child of two parents who did not have the deletion. Such new cases are known as *de novo rearrangements* or *spontaneous mutations*. This high rate of mutation, especially de novo rearrangements of the chromosome, indicated that the region of chromosome 22 represented a *hot spot*, or a highly unstable portion of the human genome prone to rearrangements. The reason for this instability is a unique evolutionary arrangement of chromosome 22 that flanks the region typically deleted in VCFS.

Chromosome 22 has a series of DNA sequences known as low copy repeats, or LCRs. Low copy repeats, also known as segmental duplications, are regions in the genome comprised of genes and also DNA sequences known as pseudogenes (segments of DNA resembling genes that do not function as genes because they do not encode for proteins) originally formed in the genome by a duplication process (Babcock et al., 2003). Chromosome 22 at q11.2 band has an apparently unique arrangement of LCRs, with multiple copies of similar or identical DNA sequences spanning a submicroscopic

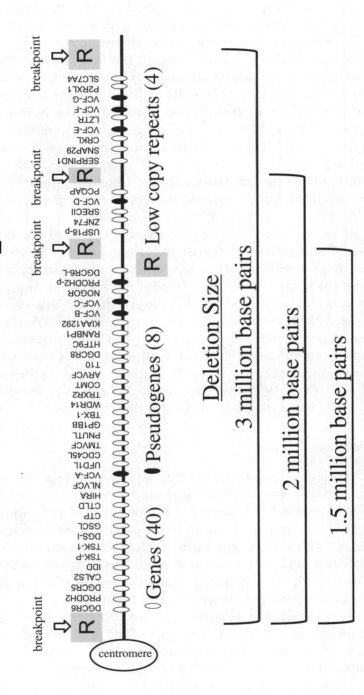

**FIGURE 3–2.** The breakpoints demonstrating the size of the deletion in chromosome 22 at the q11.2 band that causes VCFS. Note the distribution of four sets of low copy repeats (LCRs) at 22q11.2 and how they coincide with the breakpoints for the deletion of 22q11.2 found in VCFS. The genome at 22q11.2 contains 40 genes (white circles) and eight pseudogenes (black circles).

segment of the chromosome (Figure 3–2). With the proximal breakpoint the same for nearly all cases of VCFS (Morrow et al., 1995), the variation in the deletion size has been demonstrated to be caused by the location of the other LCRs that are more distal (further away from the centromere). The majority of individuals with VCFS are deleted between the first LCR and the fourth, a region that spans 3 Mb and contains 40 genes and eight pseudogenes (Figure 3–2). The presence of these LCRs explains how the deletion occurs and why the majority of the cases are new mutations. It has been found that the arrangement of these LCRs results in an abnormal recombination event during the meiotic cell divisions during the production of sperm or eggs (Edelmann et al., 1999).

In 1999, chromosome 22 became the first human chromosome to be completely sequenced, but the identification of all of the genes on chromosome 22 followed by several years. The 90% of individuals with VCFS who have the 3 Mb deletion between the first series of LCRs and the fourth (Figure 3–2) do not have a perfectly consistent phenotype. Most have congenital heart disease, but many do not. Therefore, it would seem that the size of the deletion is not solely responsible for variability of expression. Approximately 8% have deletions that cover the 1.5 Mb between the first and second series of LCRs or the 2 Mb between the first and third LCRs. The 1.5 Mb deletion encompasses 30 genes, and the 2 Mb deletion spans 34 genes. Fewer than 1% have smaller unique deletions at 22q11.2. Although it has been stated that there is no difference in expression of the syndrome based on the size of the deletion (Morrow et al., 1995), there has not really been a careful phenotypic analysis according to deletion size to confirm this hypothesis.

### How the Deletion Occurs

During the first stage of meiosis, the 46 chromosomes align side-by-side in the center of the cell that is about to divide (Figure 3–3). The 22 matching pairs of autosomes (numbered 1 through 22) and one pair of sex chromosomes (two X chromosomes in females and an X and a Y chromosome in males) line up in double file with the chromosomes in a double stranded state following replication of their DNA. The two chromosomes of each pair of autosomes get very close to each other in a stage known as synapsis. It is at this point that some DNA is exchanged between the chromosomes, a process called *crossing over* (older term) or *recombination* (newer term). Crossing over is a mechanism that is conjectured to be a part of the process of chromosome repair while also keeping the human species genetically sound by mixing segments of maternal and paternal DNA for increased variability of the genome (Figure 3–4). Crossing over tends to occur in locations within our genome where there are relatively large gaps between individual genes, as is the case in the region where the LCRs occur. When DNA is exchanged from one chromosome to another, there must be an equal exchange of genetic material.

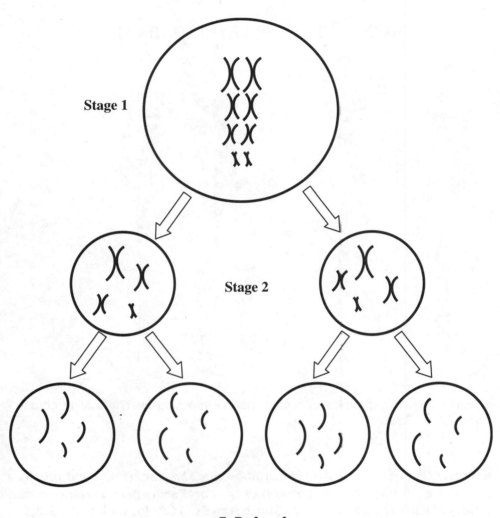

# Meiosis

**FIGURE 3–3.** Meiotic cell division showing the process by which cells go from the diploid to haploid state in an imaginary organism that has four chromosome pairs.

Specifically, the DNA from one chromosome that is switched to the other copy must contain the same genomic information. In this way, there is no loss of information from one chromosome to the other, but there is a change resulting in different versions of the genes.

The process of meiotic recombination can only be successful if the same genes are interchanged. It is therefore important that the chromosomes align in such a manner that assures the equal exchange. This relies on the DNA sequences recognizing a template for matching to the other member of the chromosome pair. The sequences within the LCR regions provide such a

# Stage 1 Meiosis (Metaphase)

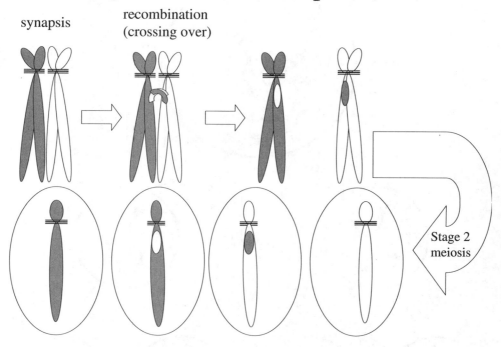

**FIGURE 3–4.** The process of recombination (crossing over) involving chromosome 22 at 22q11.2

template (Figure 3–5). However, chromosome 22 at the q11.2 band provides a challenge to this process. The copies of repeat sequences at the proximal series of LCRs are identical to the fourth series of LCRs located 3 Mb away further down the chromosome. It has been shown that an unequal exchange of chromosome material occurs when the chromosomes misalign (Edelmann et al., 1999) because the first series of LCRs recognizes the fourth series of LCRs, causing a shift in the position of the chromosomes when the recombination occurs (Figure 3–5). Therefore, one copy of the chromosome loses a piece of 22q11 while the other copy gains a piece. The resulting chromosomes will be part of an egg or sperm that may become part of a fertilized zygote resulting in either a child with VCFS (the chromosome copy that lost a piece) or a child with dup22q11 syndrome (the chromosome copy that gained a piece). VCFS is found far more frequently than dup22q11 syndrome, and this may be because dup22q11 syndrome is less compatible with long-term survival, or many fetuses with the duplication do not reach term. It is also possible that a piece of chromosome can be lost if the first set of repeats recognizes the fourth set of repeats on the same chromosome, so that it loops over on itself and splices out the intervening segment of chromosome (Figure 3–5). Because the first set of LCRs and the fourth set of LCRs on chromosome 22 are iden-

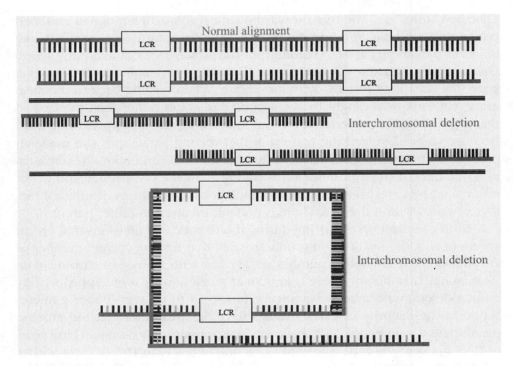

**FIGURE 3–5.** At top, the chromosomes are aligned correctly during synapsis in the first stage of meiosis as part of the normal recombination process. Below that, an error in meiotic recombination leading to a 22q11.2 deletion occurs when the recombination event is an interchromosomal error of exchange of DNA during crossing over (recombination) between the two copies of chromosome 22. The misalignment resulting in lost DNA occurs when the first series of low copy repeats aligns with the second set on its partner chromosome rather than the first. This type of error occurs in approximately 90% of cases of VCFS. At bottom, the loss of DNA occurs as a result of an intrachromosomal event where one copy of chromosome 22 loops over on itself, splicing out the 22q11.2 segment.

tical, the most common deletion occurs between these two sets of genomic sequences. However, on occasion, the deletion happens between the first and second sets of LCRs, a deletion that measures approximately 1.5 million base pairs, and even less frequently, between the first and third sets of sequences, a span of approximately 2 million base pairs. It is not clear as yet if there is any difference in the expression of the syndrome that corresponds to these three different size deletions.

When new mutations occur in a child with VCFS who has two parents who do not have the deletion, the cause is a genetic accident instigated by a misalignment of the chromosomes during meiosis. The following analogy may illustrate this point. Imagine you are reading a magazine article when something distracts you. The article you are reading is about a series of storms in Florida that caused flooding and damage to homes. When you get distracted you have just started reading a paragraph that starts with the phrase,

"The first storm . . . " You turn away from your reading for a moment and then return to the article. You find the phrase, "The first storm . . . " at the beginning of a paragraph and start reading, but the article does not make any sense. Looking over the page, you realize that there are two paragraphs on the same page that start with exactly the same phrase. When turning back to the magazine, your eye was caught by the second paragraph rather than the first so that a good deal of material key to understanding the article was not read. Because you recognized the pattern in that second paragraph, you made an error of recognition. This is essentially how the error in meiotic recombination occurs. This type of mutation is purely a chance occurrence and is not influenced by external events such as radiation, toxins, or even unusual biological states within the cell. There is no fault involved in either parent.

With the deletion occurring during the meiotic cell divisions that create sperm or ova, the result is a reproductive cell that has the correct number of chromosomes (the haploid number, or 23), but with a piece of chromosome 22 missing. This missing piece is known as a deletion, or more appropriately a microdeletion, because it is typically too small to be seen under a microscope in the majority of cases. Studies have demonstrated that the missing piece spans a segment of DNA that contains approximately 3 million base pairs of DNA in over 90% of people with VCFS, and in less than 10% of cases, either 1.5 million or 2 million base pairs. The size of the deletion corresponds to the location of the low copy repeats on chromosome 22 and the point where the error in recombination occurs.

### Identifying the Genes in the Deleted Region

Identifying genes can be done in a number of ways, and it is likely that more ways will be discovered in the future. The purpose of the Human Genome Project, completed in 2003, was to define the human genome and identify all of its genes and what they do. Although the Human Genome Project was completed when the entire human genome had been sequenced, the exact number of human genes, what they do, and how they do it is still not completely known. The process is complicated but important to understand, especially in relation to VCFS because of its large number of behavioral, learning, and psychiatric phenotypes.

One way genes are identified is by determining the starting and stopping points for the production of proteins. The protein encoding portions of genes are known as exons. Exons are packets of information within individual genes that are transcribed by RNA (mRNA), with that message being taken to the ribosomes for the production of proteins. The mRNA is translated by tRNA in the ribosomes, and that translation of the DNA sequence results in a series of codons that produce amino acids. Amino acids are strung together into polypeptide chains, and these polypeptide chains provide the basis for the proteins that do everything in our bodies. The translated code that leads to the production of an amino acid is a sequence of three nucleotides known as a codon. There are 64 codons, specific RNA sequences, that lead to the production of each amino acid. The beginning of each gene protein product is initiated by a single codon known as a start codon (the sequence of adenine, uracil, and guanine, or AUG). The end of the string of amino acids is reached when a stop codon is translated. There are three stop codons, UAG, UGA, and UAA. By scanning the genome for sequences that are translated as AUG and concluded with UAG, UGA, or UAA, all of the start and stop codons are detected that mark protein encoding portions of the genome and hence genes. The nucleotide sequences between the start and stop codons can then be sequenced to identify the chemical code of the gene.

Another way genes can be identified is to compare DNA sequences to known genes or segments of genes that produce known proteins or known traits. Looking for these sequences across the entire human genome helps to identify the exact location of the gene on one of the 23 pairs of human chromosomes.

### Determining What the Genes Do, Identifying Candidate Genes for Specific Phenotypes, and Identifying Polymorphisms

Genes perform their function by encoding for proteins. Proteins make everything in our bodies happen, from assembling us as embryos to keeping our metabolic and neurologic functions going after we are born. Genes are basically a set of encoded instructions in the nucleus of each cell that are decoded in the nucleus with a message, which leaves the nucleus and is carried to structures in the cytoplasm known as ribosomes. In the ribosomes, the genetic instructions carried by the genes are decoded further in a manner that allows a protein to be formed. That protein can remain in the cell and affect the function of the cell, or the protein can leave the cell and go elsewhere in the body to modify a structure or function distant to that cell. Because all of our cells (except eggs and sperm) have two copies of each autosome (chromosomes 1 through 22), each gene exists in two copies.

---

### *How Genes Work*

The molecule that makes life possible is DNA, deoxyribonucleic acid. Most people have some familiarity with DNA and the DNA molecule because of the many scientific reports in the news in recent history. Most people would even recognize the "double helix" structure of DNA (Figure 3–6), a discovery that would garner the Nobel Prize for James Watson and Francis Crick in 1962 based on

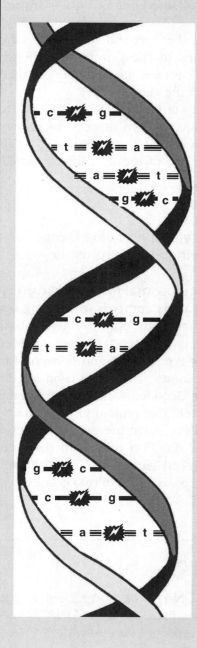

**FIGURE 3–6.** The structure of DNA. Two sugar phosphate strands are intertwined in a helix and are connected by a relatively weak electrochemical bond between organic bases. This bond, known as a base pair, along with its attached segment of the sugar phosphate backbone, is a nucleotide. The human genome contains approximately 3 billion nucleotides. Considerably less than 5% of our DNA encodes for proteins (i.e., genes).

the large body of their work in the 1950s. Our genome consists of approximately 25,000 genes. Genes are portions of DNA molecules that are strung along the chromosomes in the nuclei of our cells. DNA consists of two sugar phosphate strands that are intertwined in a helix and are connected by a relatively weak electrochemical bond between organic bases. There are four organic bases: adenine, cytosine, guanine, and thymine. Adenine can only bond with thymine, and cytosine can only bond with guanine. This bond is known as a base pair, and along with its attached segment of the sugar phosphate backbone, the unit is known as a nucleotide. It is the order and sequence of these base pairs that carry information, which must leave the nucleus of the cell in order to perform its function. The human genome contains approximately 3 billion base pairs, but considerably less than 5% of our DNA encodes for proteins. The balance of our DNA is often labeled "junk DNA." The reason why there is so much DNA that does not seem to have a specific task is not yet known.

The DNA code in the nucleus of each cell must somehow be deciphered in order to have the message transmitted to the organism. The process is performed in a number of steps (Figure 3–7); these steps require the transcription of the message in the nucleus, and the message then leaves the nucleus to be translated elsewhere so that proteins can be manufactured to perform the specific function of the gene. The first step of the process is for the base pair sequence in the genes to be transcribed. This is done by small segments of RNA, a molecule similar to DNA that has the ability to read its code. The RNA only transcribes the genetic code that encodes for proteins, and not the junk DNA. The RNA segments that transcribed the DNA code, known as mRNA or messenger RNA, are able to leave the nucleus of the cell and travel to a structure in the cell's cytoplasm known as a ribosome. In the ribosome, the mRNA has the message translated by another type of RNA, tRNA, which is capable of using the code to manufacture amino acids that are strung together in a structure known as a polypeptide chain (amino acids joined together by peptide bonds). Polypeptide chains are the structural basis for proteins. Proteins are the basis for everything that happens in embryonic development and functioning of the body after birth. The proteins produced in the ribosomes either stay within that cell to transform it or enable a particular cellular function, or leave the cell, enter the bloodstream, and carry their message to a particular organ or tissue.

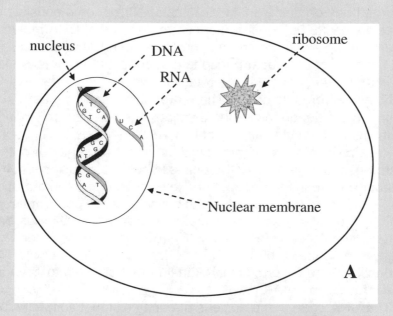

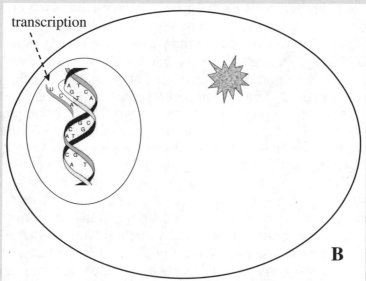

**FIGURE 3–7.** How the DNA code is transcribed and translated. (**a**) In the nucleus of the cell, a small segment of RNA known as mRNA transcribes the message from the chromosome DNA by matching its genetic code to that of the chromosome. The only difference in the code of the mRNA is that uracil replaces thymine as one of the organic bases. (**b**) The mRNA transcribes a segment of the chromosomal DNA. *continues*

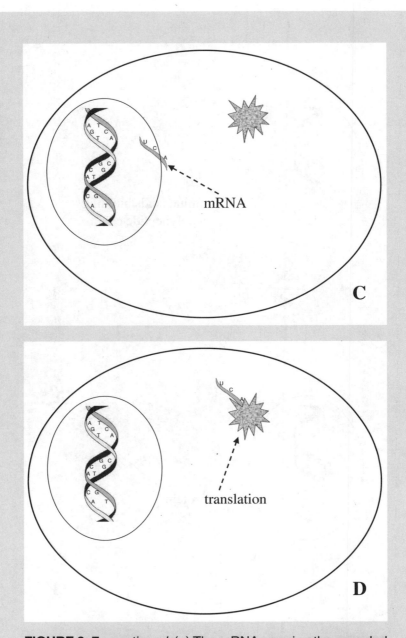

**FIGURE 3–7.** *continued* (**c**) The mRNA carrying the encoded message leaves the cell's nucleus and travels to (**d**) a ribosome in the cell's cytoplasm. There the message is translated. Another molecule of RNA, tRNA (transfer RNA), enables the codons in mRNA to be translated into the sequence of amino acids. *continues*

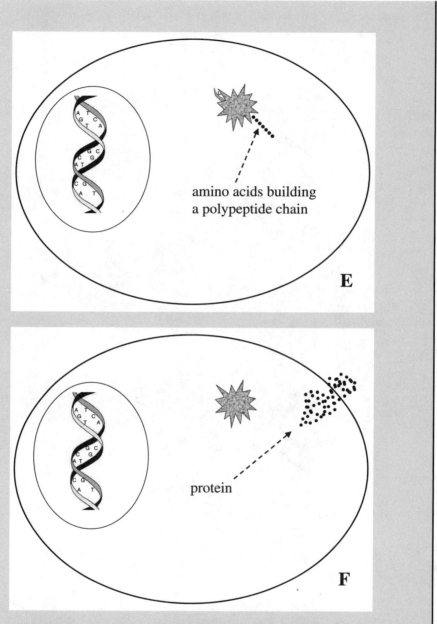

**FIGURE 3–7.** *continued*  (**e**) The amino acids are strung together to form a polypeptide chain that (**f**) forms a protein, which can leave the cell or stay within it to perform a specific function.

Genes encode for the production of proteins, and for many traits, the proper expression of that trait requires the protein from both genes. One can look at the expression of the genetic code as a sort of recipe. Like many recipes, sometimes ingredients can be altered without appreciably harming the final dish. For example, suppose you received an unexpected visit and you had to prepare dinner for your guests. You decide to make your specialty, spaghetti with marinara sauce. Your recipe calls for several pounds of fresh plum tomatoes, a bulb of garlic, a small amount of salt, some olive oil, some oregano, and two pounds of spaghetti. Your guests are on the way and you don't have time to go to the store. Several scenarios may occur:

Scenario 1: You go to your pantry and refrigerator for the ingredients and find you have everything you need. This scenario is similar to having your entire genome intact with no deletion present on chromosome 22. The result is your usual delicious sauce on enough spaghetti to serve the entire crowd.

Scenario 2: You go to your pantry and you have all of your ingredients but only half of some of them. You have all of the tomatoes and spaghetti you need, but only half of the olive oil, half of the salt, half of the garlic, and half of the oregano. You still make the sauce and it is good, although not as good as your normal recipe. But nonetheless, it is a good marinara and makes a functional meal. This is similar to the scenario for many patients with VCFS and is analogous to what happens when half of the normal complement for some genes is missing. The majority of people with VCFS have some differences from other people, yet they are nonetheless people who can do most of the things that other people do, albeit with some deficits. This is because they are missing half of the dose of certain protein products in the same way that your altered sauce has half of the garlic, salt, olive oil, and oregano.

Scenario 3: You go to your pantry and you have all of your ingredients but only half of the tomatoes and spaghetti. Now you do not have a viable meal, because the tomatoes are the single most important ingredient and one pound of spaghetti will not feed everyone. Some ingredients are critical and are needed in sufficient or exact amounts. In some cases, this also happens with VCFS, because some babies with the syndrome do not reach term or die shortly after birth from severe heart or brain anomalies. This also happens in other genetic conditions that involve deletions or alterations of genetic material. For example, in most cases of trisomy 13 or trisomy 18, children do not survive to term or die shortly after birth.

As the scenarios above demonstrate, the genome is a well-balanced recipe. When all genes are present in the normal diploid number, the variations in the recipe (allelic variations) are those that result in the normal variations in human form and behavior that are not considered abnormal, such as blue eyes versus brown eyes, or normal versus superior intellect. Such variations are caused by different versions of genes, known as alleles or polymorphisms. It is, therefore, the deficiency in certain protein products of one or more of the deleted genes that results in the problems expressed by people with VCFS.

Determining what the genes in the deleted region do when so many genes are deleted is a challenge. With over 180 anomalies being documented

---

### Genetic Variation: Alleles and Polymorphisms

All people have the same number of genes. In fact, within a species, all members of that species share the same basic genome. Each gene in an individual human has a corresponding gene that performs the same function in every other person. However, genes for a particular function come in a number of different versions. Models of cars would be an apt analogy. Automobiles are all basically the same in that they perform the same function. They have wheels, steering wheels, windshields, engines, brakes, and so on. However, there are many different types of cars. There are Ford Mustangs and Rolls Royce Phantoms, Jeep Wranglers and Cadillac limousines. Genes are the same in that all people have genes for eye color, but minor differences in those genes result in a variety of eye colors, from blue to brown. These different versions of genes are known as *alleles*. The term *polymorphism* refers to the presence of two or more alleles of a gene within a species. When a variation in the DNA sequences of a gene occurs in less than 1% of the population, it is considered to be a mutation, whether deleterious or advantageous. Polymorphisms in genes within the 22q11.2 region may be important in VCFS. Because one copy of each gene within the 22q11.2 region is present on the normal copy of chromosome 22, the expression of that version of the gene may cause variations in expression of the syndrome. It is known that a mutation of the gene *GP1BB* (glycoprotein Ib, a platelet surface membrane glycoprotein) can cause Bernard-Soulier syndrome, a severe bleeding disorder, when that mutation is present in someone with VCFS who is missing a normal copy of *GP1BB* (Budarf et al., 1995). It is also possible for certain alleles to afford a protection against certain diseases. Therefore, understanding the function of all of the deleted genes plus knowing all of the polymorphisms is critical to understanding how VCFS is expressed and why there is such significant variability of expression.

in VCFS and 40 genes deleted in the 3 Mb deletion, the number of possible combinations in genotype to phenotype correlation is obviously large. Gene effects are often pleiotropic, meaning that they can affect more than one organ, system, or function. Therefore, it is possible that the effects seen in people with VCFS may be related to relatively few of the deleted genes. Of course, it is also possible that each gene plays a role. Complicating issues further is the fact that genes often regulate or influence other genes (known as downstream regulation) or genes may be regulated by other genes elsewhere in the genome (upstream regulation). Gene-to-gene interactions are now being studied in VCFS, and several such interactions have already been identified. Two genes have been found to interact with *TBX1*, the gene that is responsible for the heart anomalies in VCFS (Merscher et al., 2001). A gene labeled *VEGF* (vascular endothelial growth factor) interacts with *TBX1* and has been implicated in the phenotype of VCFS (Moon et al., 2006; Stalmans et al., 2003). Another homeobox gene, *PITX2*, is regulated downstream by *TBX1* (Nowotschin et al., 2006). Inactivation of *VEGF* results in many vascular and cardiovascular anomalies, while loss of function of *PITX2* results in body symmetry abnormalities as well as heart malformations. *TBX1* may also regulate fibroblast growth factor genes, *FGF8* and *FGF10* (Hu et al., 2004; Vitelli, Taddei, Morishima, Meyers, & Baldini, 2002; Xu et al., 2004). *FGF* genes are also important to embryonic development.

### Animal Models and Knockouts

One way to identify what genes do is to see their effects in animal models and then to manipulate the genomes of those animals to see the effects of changes in their genome. When individual genes or groups of genes are inactivated in an animal model, this genomic manipulation is known as a *knockout*, and the mouse is typically used as a model for study.

Animals, especially other mammals, can be used in this type of experiments because the genomes of most animal species are very similar. In fact, the mouse shares almost all of our genes. The human and mouse genomes each have approximately three billion base pairs of DNA, approximately the same number of genes, and similar distributions of those genes over their chromosomes (40 for the mouse, 46 in humans). In the case of VCFS, mouse chromosome 16 contains a region that is homologous (nearly identical) to chromosome 22 in the human, sharing almost all of the genes at 22q11.2. Although there are several novel genes in the human 22q11 compared to mouse chromosome 16, a majority of the genes at 22q11.2 are present in the mouse in the same order as on human chromosome 22.

Using a knockout mouse model, a major breakthrough in understanding how the deletion causes some of the anomalies in VCFS was made (Merscher et al., 2001). Deletion of the gene *TBX1* was identified as the cause of the heart anomalies in VCFS. *TBX1*, usually referred to as T-Box 1, belongs to a class of genes (T-Box) that are transcription factors responsible for embryonic developmental processes. The deletion from chromosome 22 that causes VCFS always includes *TBX1*. Deletion of one copy of *TBX1* in the mouse causes the same heart anomalies found in humans with VCFS (Merscher et al., 2001. It is also possible that other structural anomalies in VCFS such as ear, kidney, and thymus anomalies may also be related to hemizygosity of *TBX1*, although this has not yet been proven conclusively.

Does this information about *TBX1* have any practical implications? Not at this time. Heart formation happens very early in embryogenesis, and the anomalies commonly found in VCFS are already in progress by the time many women find out that they are pregnant. Septation of the heart and formation of most of its major components are already largely completed, and the heart is beating between 4 and 5 weeks after fertilization. Therefore, at this time, correcting or reversing the action of the gene is not possible. In any event, surgery is highly effective in resolving congenital heart malformations, and the majority of infants with VCFS who have congenital heart disease survive early heart surgery without many adverse consequences. However, it is possible that the information about the role of *TBX1* will lead to major treatment advances in the future.

Other genes are being studied in addition to *TBX1* with special scrutiny of genes that are highly expressed in the brain or genes that have functions related to brain chemistry. A gene that has garnered a great deal of attention is *COMT*, cathechol-o-methyltransferase. *COMT* is responsible for degrading (catabolizing) catecholamines. Catecholamines include dopamine, epinephrine, and norepinephrine. Although these three chemical compounds circulate in the bloodstream throughout the body, they are of primary interest because of their role as neural transmitters. If one copy of *COMT* is missing, as it is in VCFS, then there is less of the protein available that is encoded for degrading dopamine and eliminating it from the brain's synapses. Elevated dopamine levels have been implicated in a number of psychiatric illnesses including bipolar disorder, schizophrenia, and ADD/ADHD (Cook et al., 1995; Diehl & Gershon, 1992; Kahn & Davis, 1995). There are several different *COMT* alleles including two polymorphisms that have large differences in the amount of dopamine that can be metabolized (Lachman et al., 1996). One version of *COMT* is the *COMT158^{met}* allele, and the other is the *COMT158^{val}* allele. These two versions are caused by a change of base pairs at codon 158 in the *COMT* gene that changes the amino acid methionine (met) to valine (val). The val allele is a high activity version of *COMT* that degrades much more dopamine than the low activity met allele. People with VCFS are missing one copy of the *COMT* gene because *COMT* is always deleted in the syndrome. Therefore, only one copy of the gene is available to deactivate dopamine in the brain's synapses. The val allele degrades approximately four times as much dopamine as the met allele. Therefore, individuals with VCFS who have only one copy of the met allele may be more likely to express mental illness than those with one copy of the val allele (Gothelf et al., 2007; Graf et al., 2001; Lachman et al., 1996). In this case, this particular knowledge could have major treatment implications if a medication were available to take over the function of the missing copy of the *COMT* allele. Three reports, all anecdotal cases or series of cases, have been published to show promising treatment effects with the drugs metyrosine or methyldopa (Caradang & Scholten, 2007; Graf et al., 2001; O'Hanlon, Ritchie, Smith, & Patel, 2003). Both of these medications are antihypertensives that act to degrade the dopamine molecule in order to reduce blood pressure. Metyrosine is used specifically to do this in individuals who have a rare adrenal tumor known as a pheochromocytoma. Pheochromocytoma is a benign tumor of the adrenal medulla that causes an oversecretion of catecholamines. Prior to surgical correction, metyrosine is given to reduce the catecholamine levels. Excessive dopamine will also elevate blood pressure because dopamine, epinephrine, and norepinephrine also have the job of regulating the amount of muscular tension in the blood vessels, thereby affecting blood pressure. Because dopamine has its highest level of activity in the brain, giving metyrosine to someone with VCFS should lower dopaminergic activity, and this has in fact been demonstrated in a small series of cases (Graf et al., 2001).

Methyldopa (also known as alpha-methyldopa and L-α-methyldopa) is also an antihypertensive that has been used for more than 40 years, most commonly known by its brand name Aldomet. Methyldopa acts in a slightly different manner, but with the same effect of lowering dopaminergic activity (O'Hanlon et al., 2003). In the case of both metyrosine and methyldopa, the attempt is to use information obtained from the genome to guide the management of presenting symptoms based on laboratory research on genomic effects. Often called "translational research," this kind of response to genomic information holds great promise in the future and should encourage continued work to decipher the effects of the deletion.

### How Is a Deletion Different from Other Types of Mutations?

Using the analogy presented earlier in this chapter of a recipe, the method of how genomic alterations result in problems needs to be addressed specifically to that problem. Identifying the genes in the deleted 22q11.2 region is not sufficient to understand the expression of phenotypes. In the case of a deletion, there is reduced dosage of the gene's activity (protein production). In trisomies or partial trisomies, there is overexpression of the involved genes, as would be the case in Down syndrome, 22q11.2 duplication, and trisomy 13. In looking at deletions and duplications of the same area of the genome, such as 22q11.2, one would broadly expect the same organs and systems to be affected because the same genes are involved. Indeed, in animal experiments, this has been found to be true (Funke, Pandita, & Morrow, 2001; Merscher et al., 2001). In reported cases of 22q11.2 duplication in humans, congenital heart disease and developmental delay were among the most common of clinical findings in affected individuals, although the range of expression is quite variable and the number of reported cases remains small.

In cases with deletions from 22q11.2 who therefore have VCFS, there is more than one possibility in terms of how abnormalities may be expressed. One possibility, and the most obvious, is that a reduction in gene dosage causes a problem with embryonic development or ongoing function because there is half the amount of protein being produced by the gene. There is clearly very good evidence for this in the expression of *TBX1* because experimental evidence in a mouse model demonstrates that loss of one copy of the gene causes the same heart anomalies as seen in humans with VCFS (Merscher et al., 2001). However, the process is clearly not as linear as one might expect because congenital heart disease is not present in all people with 22q11.2 deletions. At least 25% of people with VCFS have no heart anomalies, and this significant number demonstrates that there must be more to the abnormal development of the heart than simply loss of function of one copy of *TBX1*.

Another possible model is that the loss of one gene unmasks an abnormal effect from a single copy of the remaining gene on the normal chromosome 22. This phenomenon has been observed and reported in relation to Bernard-Soulier syndrome, which is caused by a rare mutation of one copy of the *GP1Bβ* gene that is involved in the formation of platelet surface protein. The recessive version of this gene would not normally be expressed if the normal copy of the gene were present on the other chromosome 22. However, the deletion results in the absence of a normal allele to counteract the recessive mutation, and the single abnormal copy of the gene is therefore expressed. If the copy of the *GP1Bβ* gene on the normal chromosome is not the mutated version, then most people with VCFS would have borderline normal or mild thrombocytopenia without the bleeding problems found in Bernard-Soulier syndrome. It is not yet know if there are other rare mutations or polymorphisms of genes residing on the normal copy of chromosome 22 that would be expressed as an anomaly or behavioral disorder because of the deletion.

Still another possibility is that there are genes within the 22q11.2 region that have regulatory functions or interact with genes elsewhere in the genome to perform certain functions. It is already known that *TBX1* regulates or influences other gene expressions, including *VEGF*, *PITX2*, and a number of fibroblast growth factor genes (Aggarwal et al., 2006; Nowotschin et al., 2006; Stalmans et al., 2003). It is possible that the degree or type of interaction with genes elsewhere in the genome is related to the specific polymorphism located on the normal copy of chromosome 22, or that the interaction is altered by dosage.

## Genetic Effects Outside of the 22q11.2 Region that Contribute to the Phenotype

With approximately 25,000 genes in the human genome, the number of possible interactions with genes in the deleted region are astronomically large and complicated. Intensive study of large numbers of subjects to reach the appropriate conclusions will be required. For physical and structural anomalies, animal models will be helpful, but for behavioral problems, the process is highly dependent on the study of human subjects. To emphasize the complexity of the problem, there are 190 separate anomalies listed in Chapter 2 that have been reported to be associated with VCFS. These occur because of 40 genes deleted from chromosome 22. This means a possible interaction effect that could be as complicated as 7480 possible effects of the deletion if there is a direct relationship between the deleted gene and the anomaly. Adding interactions with other genes outside of 22q11.2, such as *VEGF*, *PITX2*, *FGF8*, and *FGF10*, would increase those possibilities by many thousands. It is also possible that some of the uncommon anomalies reported in children with VCFS are not a part of the syndrome, but related to mutations elsewhere in the genome that occur coincidentally with the deletion. For uncommon anomalies, it will be important to study large numbers of cases of VCFS, which will allow clinicians to determine the true frequency of rare anomalies. Microarray analysis will help to unlock these mysteries and is now being applied to the study of VCFS in a number of studies.

It has been hypothesized that one of the major differences between humans and other species is that the human genome has more gene-to-gene interaction (upstream and downstream regulation). Although the number of genes in the human genome is not dramatically different from other species, such as the mouse, some scientists believe that part of the evolutionary process is that more complex traits can be expressed when genes are able to influence other genes. The result may be more complex protein combinations that influence the complexity of traits, including human behavior. At the present time, a substantial amount of research involving VCFS is focusing on these gene-to-gene interactions.

## Epigenetic Factors that Might Contribute to the Phenotypic Spectrum

Epigenetic factors are modifications of genes that do not change the DNA sequence (base pair arrangements) but alter the DNA molecule. A commonly observed example is the addition of methyl groups to the DNA backbone (Figure 3–8). Although the DNA code is unchanged, the addition of this group of three hydrogen atoms bonded to a carbon atom alters the ability of a gene to be transcribed properly, thereby affecting the RNA that carries information from the nucleus to the ribosome. These types of transcription errors often result in how genes get switched on and off during crucial times of embryonic development. The presence or absence of methyl groups on DNA molecules is often used by cells to differentiate between genes derived from paternal or maternal DNA. If the segment of DNA containing a particular gene is modified with methyl groups not typically present, the cell may decide to create a set of proteins from only a paternally or maternally inherited gene,

# DNA

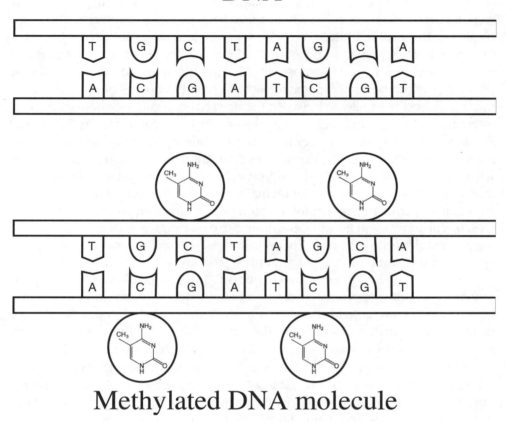

## Methylated DNA molecule

**FIGURE 3–8.** Methylation of DNA (epigenetics).

therefore resulting in different expressions of a trait depending on the parent of origin for the DNA. This phenomenon is known as imprinting and is a well-known cause of differing expressions of deletions, depending on the parent of origin for the missing DNA. Probably the best-known example of imprinting is the differing expressions of deletions from 15q11–13. When the deletion is derived from paternal DNA, the clinical manifestation is Prader-Willi syndrome, a disorder marked by developmental delay, severe hypotonia, and severe overeating in childhood resulting in morbid obesity. However, when the deletion is derived from maternal DNA, the clinical expression is Angelman syndrome, a completely different disorder with severe neurological impairment and progressive ataxia. In the case of Prader-Willi syndrome, the disorder is caused by the absence of specific paternal genes within the deleted region, while in Angelman syndrome, it is the absence of specific but different maternal genes that also reside in the deleted region. At this point, it does not appear that imprinting plays a major role if any in VCFS.

# GENETIC COUNSELING FOR VCFS

The issue of genetic counseling is different for parents of a child with VCFS than it is for a person who has VCFS. Parents of children with VCFS who do not have the syndrome themselves do not have an increased risk for having another child with the syndrome unless they have a germline mosaicism involving chromosome 22, something that is very rare. However, counseling someone who has VCFS presents a difficult case because of the difficulty in grasping certain concepts, especially those that involve thinking into the future.

The majority of people who present for genetic counseling in relation to VCFS are unaffected parents or unaffected siblings. This is because at least 90% of cases of VCFS are de novo rearrangements (new mutations). In most clinical settings, parents of children with VCFS have FISH or other molecular genetics studies done on themselves to rule out the possibility that one of them is affected. If laboratory studies confirm that neither parent is affected, it is not necessary to test their other unaffected children. Two unaffected parents means that the affected child is a new mutation, and there is no known genetic link between the copies of chromosome 22 in the parents and unaffected siblings. Therefore, the risk for future pregnancies for the parents and unaffected siblings, aunts, uncles, cousins, and all other relatives is 1:2000, the same as in the general population. It is important to explain to parents about chromosomes, DNA deletions from chromosomes, how deletions can cause problems, how the deletion occurs in VCFS, and recurrence risk for all parties involved. Autosomal dominant inheritance needs to be explained in relation to the child who is affected. The genome in the deleted region should be explained in appropriate terms for those being counseled. Of course, depending on the age of the child, one must provide caveats in relation to the potential for new discoveries in the field of genetics, both in terms of diagnosis and treatment. Some counselors provide information regarding treatment, but this should be done with caution because genetic counselors or clinical geneticists may not necessarily be aware of all treatment options for a disorder as complicated as VCFS. VCFS care often involves surgery, pharmaceuticals, speech therapy, dental treatment, and educational accommodations. Unless the counselor is very familiar with all of these issues, specifics about treatment should be avoided.

Our experience in following many families for more than 30 years has allowed us to observe the changes that have occurred in the perception of risk by parents of children with VCFS and how the discoveries described in this chapter, including the discovery of the deletion, the characterization of the deletion, FISH, and the mechanism of the deletion, have translated directly to patient care and decision making for parents of children with VCFS. To date, we have been directly or indirectly involved in the care of more than 1600 families with VCFS who have provided us with information relating to their family structure. In the early years of following families with an affected child, we found that if a child with VCFS was born into the family as the first child, the large majority of these families decided not to have more children. When the child with VCFS was born as a second or third child into a family, he was typically the last child born. Prior to the point when the deletion that causes VCFS became known to us, we were following 128 families that had a child with VCFS. More than 50% of those children were only children, and in almost every other case, the child with VCFS was the last child born into the family. In these cases, it is impossible to know how many of these parents ceased having children because their last child had VCFS. However, since 1999 (when we learned the mechanism for the deletion and were able to counsel families accordingly), we have not found this same proportion of children with VCFS being only children, and we have many instances of parents with one or more children in the family following the birth of a child with VCFS. There has been an immediate translation of information obtained from the laboratory to the counseling situation, and this affects the lives of parents of children with VCFS and their families.

## MOSAICISM AND GERMLINE (GONADAL) MOSAICISM

As with almost everything in life, there is always a loophole or exception. Mosaicism or germline mosaicism (sometimes called gonadal mosaicism) is unusual presentations that may result in multiple affected children from unaffected parents. There has been one report of an apparently unaffected mother who had two affected children with VCFS, with subsequent FISH studies on more than 150 cells showing that 7% of her lymphocytes showed the deletion (Kasprzak et al., 1998). Although the children's cases were described in detail with photographs, the mother's case was not but was described as normal. FISH was also done on the father and did not show a deletion. In mosaicisms, the mutation (deletion) occurs some time after fertilization so that only a percentage of cells are affected. Mosaicisms are common in Turner syndrome and Down syndrome. The fewer cells that have the mutation, the milder the expression.

In germline mosaicisms, the parent has a rearrangement of 22q11.2 that occurs in the cells of the testes or ovaries, which mature into reproductive cells, but the rest of the cells in the body are normal. Therefore, if a parent with a germline mosaicism has a child with VCFS that is confirmed by FISH, and the parent has FISH done to check for the deletion, the test will come back normal. This is because FISH is performed on peripheral blood samples, and the cells used for the chromosome preparation are white blood cells. The parent has the mutation only in the cells of the reproductive organs, making the chromosome rearrangement tissue-specific. The parent is unaffected by the syndrome (because the overwhelming majority of cells in the body are normal) but is still at risk for having another child with VCFS. Germline mosaicisms are often expressed when normal parents have more than one child with VCFS. Because it is known that VCFS is inherited and expressed in an autosomal dominant manner, this could only happen if the mosaicism exists. Germline mosaicism has been reported in two siblings with VCFS who have normal parents (Sandrin-Garcia et al., 2002). It is possible that there are more cases of germline mosaicism that have not been detected in situations where there is only a single affected child from a parent with a germline mosaicism. In such cases, it would be presumed that the child had a spontaneous mutation, and FISH results on the parents would not be positive for the deletion.

## COUNSELING FOR PEOPLE WITH VCFS

There are significant challenges in the process of providing genetic counseling for individuals with VCFS, as is also the case for counseling of other types. Obstacles include their cognitive abilities, difficulties with executive functioning, and putting concepts involving time and space into a realistic context. The majority of people with VCFS have very concrete thought processes and learn best by repetition and rote memorization. Problem-solving skills are impaired, and the more abstract problems become, the more difficult they are for people with VCFS. Issues related to genetics, inheritance, consequences of sexual activity in terms of reproduction, and putting the raising of a child into proper perspective are extremely difficult for a person with VCFS. People with VCFS are often impulsive and may respond more readily to immediate needs and feelings than things they have been taught by their parents. The specifics of recurrence risk that would be discussed in a counseling session may not be remembered at a specific moment in the future for a person with VCFS, and judgment may be overshadowed by more elemental urges. For example, sexual urges may not be well understood. The desire to have a baby may be reinforced by an idealized but unrealistic picture of how VCFS might play a role in child rearing. This is not to say that people with VCFS cannot or should not have children, or that people with VCFS would make bad parents. Each case needs to be evaluated individually according to the specific situation, the total family and support network, and level of functioning. There are many people with VCFS who are parents and who are very good parents, while others are mentally and cognitively impaired to the point they cannot manage their children appropriately.

Counseling sessions need to be different for people who have VCFS. For one thing, sessions should be repeated more than once. People close to the affected person, such as parents, spouses, siblings, or friends, should be brought into the session and be given as much information as possible in writing and pictorial form. Figure 3–9 (located on enclosed DVD as a slide presentation) consists of a series of pictures used at the VCFS International Center at Upstate Medical University for counseling, demonstrating a picture of chromosomes, a FISH study, the genes on the chromosome, a pictorial representation of mei-otic recombination, and the mechanism for the deletion. The pictures are all captioned to explain the process that causes the deletion. These are reviewed with the person receiving counseling and with others who can help to rein-force information discussed during the session.

It is also important to use words and concrete language and examples that can be understood by people with VCFS. If medical or scientific terms need to be used, they should be explained in ways that make them easily under-stood. For example, the analogy of a recipe described earlier in this chapter can be used to explain DNA and genes. Other familiar examples can be used, but the important thing is that the explanation should be tailored to the patient and his level of understanding, not the counselor's. Follow-up contacts should be scheduled periodically to assure the efficacy of the session.

Although complicated, understanding the genetics of VCFS provides a powerful learning tool for a large number of genetic disorders, and more importantly, for common disorders such as psychiatric illness, speech and lan-guage impairment, learning disabilities, ADD/ADHD, and autism spectrum dis-order. Continued study of VCFS may lead to understanding of the mechanisms that cause these disorders and therefore point towards effective treatments.

# REFERENCES

Aggarwall, V. S., Liao, J., Bondarev, A., Schimmang, T., Lewandoski, M., Locker, J., et al. (2006). Dissection of Tbx1 and Fgf interactions in mouse models of 22q11DS sug-gests functional redundancy. *Human Molecular Genetics, 15,* 3219–3228.

Babcock, M., Pavlicek, A., Spiteri, E., Kashork, C. D., Ioshikhes, I., Shaffer, L. G. (2003). Shuffling of genes within low-copy repeats on 22q11 (LCR22) by Alu-mediated recombination events during evolution. *Genome Research, 13,* 2519-2532.

Budarf, M. L., Konkle, B. A., Ludlow, L. B., Michaud, D., Yamashiro, D. J., McDonald McGinn, D., et al. (1995). Identification of a patient with Bernard-Soulier syndrome and a deletion in the DiGeorge/velo-cardio-facial chromosomal region in 22q11.2. *Human Molecular Genetics, 4,* 763–766.

Carandang, C. G., & Scholten, M. C. (2007). Metyrosine in psychosis associated with 22q11.2 deletion syndrome: Case report. *Journal of Child and Adolescent Psycho-pharmacology, 17,* 115–120.

Cook, E. H., Stein, M. A., Krasowski, M. D., Cox, N. J., Olken, D. M., Kieffer, J. E., et al. (1995). Association of attention deficit disorder and the dopamine transporter gene. *American Journal of Human Genetics, 56,* 993–998.

Diehl, D. J., & Gershon, S. (1992). The role of dopamine in mood disorders. *Compre-hensive Psychiatry, 33,* 115–120.

Edelmann, L., Pandita, R. K., Spiteri, E., Funke, B., Goldberg, R., Palanisamy, N., et al. (1999). A common molecular basis for rearrangement disorders on chromosome 22q11. *Human Molecular Genetics, 8,* 1157–1167.

Funke, B., Pandita, R. K., & Morrow, B. E. (2001). Isolation and characterization of a novel gene containing WD40 repeats from the region deleted in velo-cardio-facial/DiGeorge syndrome on chromosome 22q11. *Genomics, 73*, 264–271.

Gothelf, D., Feinstein, C., Thompson, T., Gu, E., Penniman, L., Van Stone, E., et al. (2007). Risk factors for the emergence of psychotic disorders in adolescents with 22q11.2 deletion syndrome. *American Journal of Psychiatry, 164*, 663–669

Graf, W. D., Unis, A. S., Yates, C. M., Sulzbacher, S., Dinulos, M. B., Jack, R. M., et al. (2001). Catecholamines in patients with 22q11.2 deletion syndrome and the low-activity *COMT* polymorphism. *Neurology, 57*, 410–416.

Hill, A. S., Foot, N. J., Chaplin, T. L., & Young, C. D. (2000). The most frequent constitutional translocation in humans, the t(11;22)(q23;q11), is due to a highly specific Alu-mediated recombination. *Human Molecular Genetics, 9*, 1523–1532.

Hu, T., Yamagishi, H., Maeda, J., McAnally, J., Yamagishi, C., & Srivastava, D. (2004). Tbx1 regulates fibroblast growth factors in the anterior heart field through a reinforcing autoregulatory loop involving forkhead transcription factors. *Development, 131*, 5491–5502.

Kahn, R. S., & Davis, K. L. (1995). New developments in dopamine and schizophrenia. In F. Bloom & D. Kupfer (Eds.), *Psychopharmacology: The fourth generation of progress* (pp. 1193–1203). New York: Raven Press.

Kasprzak, L., Der Kaloustian, V. M., Elliott, A. M., Shevell, M., Lejtenyi, C., & Eydoux, P. (1998). Deletion of 22q11 in two brothers with different phenotype. *American Journal of Medical Genetics, 75*, 288–291.

Lachman, H. M., Morrow, B., Shprintzen, R. J., Veit, S., Parsia, S. S., Faedda, G., et al. (1996). Association of codon 108/158 catechol-o-methyl transferase gene polymorphism with the psychiatric manifestations of VCFS. *American Journal of Medical Genetics, 67*, 468–472.

Merscher, S., Funke, B., Epstein, J. A., Heyer, J., Puech, A., Lu, M. M., et al. (2001). TBX1 is responsible for cardiovascular defects in velo-cardio-facial/DiGeorge syndrome. *Cell, 104*, 619–629.

Moon, A. M., Guris, D. L., Seo, J. H., Li, L., Hammond, J, Talbot, A., et al. (2006). Crkl deficiency disrupts Fgf8 signaling in a mouse model of 22q11 deletion syndromes. *Developmental Cell, 10*, 71–80.

Morrow, B., Goldberg, R., Carlson, C., Gupta, R. D., Sirotkin, H., Collins, J., et al. (1995). Molecular definition of the 22q11 deletions in velo-cardio-facial syndrome. *American Journal of Human Genetics, 56*, 1391–1403.

Nowotschin, S., Liao, J., Gage, P. J., Epstein, J. A., Campione, M., & Morrow, B. E. (2006). Tbx1 affects asymmetric cardiac morphogenesis by regulating *Pitx2* in the secondary heart field. *Development, 133*, 1565–1573.

O'Hanlon, J. F., Ritchie, R. C., Smith, E. A., & Patel, R. (2003). Replacement of antipsychotic and antiepileptic medication by L-alpha-methyldopa in a woman with velo-cardiofacial syndrome. *International Clinical Psychopharmacology, 18*, 117–119.

Sandrin-Garcia, P., Macêdo, C., Martelli, L. R., Ramos, E. S., Guion-Almeida, M. L., Richieri-Costa, A. et al. (2002). Recurrent 22q11.2 deletion in a sibship suggestive of parental germline mosaicism in velocardiofacial syndrome. *Clinical Genetics, 61*, 380–383.

Scambler, P. J., Kelly, D., Lindsay, E., Williamson, R., Goldberg, R., Shprintzen, R. J., et al. (1992). Velo-cardio-facial syndrome associated with chromosome 22 deletions encompassing the DiGeorge locus. *Lancet, 339*, 1138–1139.

Shprintzen, R. J., Goldberg, R. B., Lewin, M. L., Sidoti, E. J., Berkman, M. D., Argamaso, R. V., et al. (1978). A new syndrome involving cleft palate, cardiac anomalies, typical facies, and learning disabilities: Velo-cardio-facial syndrome. *Cleft Palate Journal*, *15*, 56–62.

Shprintzen, R. J., Goldberg, R., Young, D., & Wolford, L. (1981). The velo-cardio-facial syndrome: A clinical and genetic analysis. *Pediatrics*, *67*, 167–172.

Stalmans, I., Lambrechts, D., De smet, F., Jansen, S., Wang, J., Maity, S., et al. (2003). VEGF: A modifier of the del22q11 (DiGeorge) syndrome? *Nature Medicine*, *9*, 173–182.

Williams, M. A., Shprintzen, R. J., & Goldberg, R. B. (1985). Male-to-male transmission of the velo-cardio-facial syndrome: A case report and review of 60 cases. *Journal of Craniofacial and Genetic Development Biology*, *5*, 175–180.

Vitelli, F., Taddei, I., Morishima, M., Meyers, E. N., & Baldini, A. (2002). A genetic link between Tbx1 and fibroblast growth factor signaling. *Development*, *129*, 4605–4611.

Xu, H., Morishima, M., Wylie, J. N., Schwartz, R. J., Bruneau, B. G., Lindsay, E. A., et al. (2004). Tbx1 has a dual role in the morphogenesis of the cardiac outflow tract. *Development*, *131*, 3217–3227.

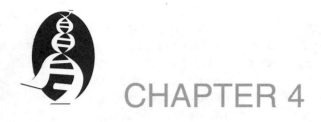

# CHAPTER 4

# Triage in VCFS: Utilizing the Natural History

*I*t is common for people to wonder if having a diagnosis such as VCFS is helpful or if it "labels" children or adults in a manner that stigmatizes them and perhaps defines them in a way that is counterproductive. Although there may be some negative ramifications of being identified with a "disease" that has both cognitive and mental problems as key features, there is one overriding reason for having the diagnosis. As has been pointed out in the earliest days of the fields of dysmorphology, clinical genetics, and syndromology, syndromic diagnosis reveals three key elements that are vital to good patient care. They are the syndrome's phenotypic spectrum, its natural history, and the prognosis (Shprintzen, 1997). Phenotypic spectrum refers to all of the anomalies associated with a disorder that have been observed by the examiner, reported in the literature, or are commonly known as clinical features. Knowing the phenotypic spectrum of a disorder allows clinicians to anticipate that certain anomalies may be present that may not be obvious unless specifically assessed. For example, renal anomalies are relatively common in VCFS, often unilateral, and most often asymptomatic. Renal ultrasound will reveal these anomalies, but renal ultrasound is not a typical examination for most people until some type of genitourinary symptom is detected. If one knew the phenotypic spectrum of VCFS as described in detail in Chapter 2, renal ultrasound would be scheduled routinely for all patients with VCFS.

Natural history refers to the course of the syndrome over time. Many anomalies in VCFS are not present at birth, and some that are present may disappear later or progress and become worse over time. It is therefore important to know how to schedule assessments in the future for people with VCFS. This type of time-sensitive management is important to intercept problems and to prevent them from becoming issues that impair quantity or quality of life. In some cases, issues presenting early in life that might seem to require aggressive management actually may not because they become less problematic over time. For example, growth and weight gain can be poor in infants with VCFS, and this may prompt management of feeding problems by surgical means, such as gastrostomy or gavage feeding. However, if it is known that feeding and growth are not strongly related in VCFS and that the natural history of growth is different in VCFS than in normal children, such aggressive steps might not be taken. This issue will be discussed in detail in Chapter 5.

Prognosis is, of course, important in knowing how treatments turn out and how much effort should be expended in certain areas of care. If the prognosis in certain areas of need is excellent, then one would want to apply all appropriate therapies to alleviate the problem. Prognosis is of particular importance in terms of education and learning for children with VCFS. Will a child with VCFS be able to grasp complicated issues related to mathematics? Will she be able to solve algebraic problems? If most children with VCFS have severe problems with these issues, should they be placed in a class where the curriculum is not specifically suited to this weakness?

In this chapter, a general plan of management will be laid out that takes into account the phenotypic spectrum of the syndrome, its natural history, and long-term prognosis. The reasons for these suggestions relate to all of the issues discussed in Chapter 2. The specific evaluations will be listed alphabetically with proposed schedules for each assessment. Of course, the need for these assessments requires the appropriate personnel and skill sets to implement them. One of the challenges in obtaining health care and long-term management for children with VCFS is the need to have multiple specialists with specific knowledge about VCFS and then having someone who knows how to tie all of the different components together into a cohesive treatment plan. We will not adress educational assessments in this chapter in part because of the excellent text by Donna Cutler-Landsman (2007) that addresses these aspects in great detail. We can say, however, that nearly all children with VCFS require educational assessments and these should begin at the earliest possible opportunity on entering school.

## AUDIOLOGY (HEARING TESTING)

Although many children have newborn hearing screening by otoacoustic emissions (OAE) or auditory brainstem response (ABR), these tests are meant to identify gross problems with hearing. False positives and false negatives can occur with newborn screenings, so a more informative hearing test is recommended. The specific administration of these tests may depend on the age at which the diagnosis of VCFS is made or the motor development of the child. In newborns and young infants, it is necessary to use electrophysiological tests such as brainstem audiometry to identify hearing loss, but as the child approaches the first birthday, it may be possible to get an accurate behavioral test using play audiometry. In older children and adults, threshold testing is performed using behavioral audiometry, in which individuals being tested are instructed to respond to sounds they hear administered at a variety of hearing levels. Included in this battery of tests should be speech audiometry, in which patients are asked to repeat words that they hear at varying sound levels. In addition to testing hearing sensitivity, speech audiometry can provide some information about speech perception. Tympanometry is another type of electrophysiologic test that involves the measurement of resistance or impedance of the eardrum (tympanic membrane) and the bones of the middle ear to pressure induced in the outer ear canal. It is a test of middle ear function, not hearing sensitivity. Because children with VCFS often have fluid in the middle ear, they will typically require frequent tympanometry tests. Middle ear fluid causes the eardrum to be less compliant and more resistant to pressure, and this can be detected by tympanometry.

Another audiometric assessment is of auditory processing, often referred to as central auditory processing, or CAP. ABR, OAE, play audiometry, and behavioral threshold testing assess hearing sensitivity. CAP testing is designed to assess what the brain does with what we hear (Katz, 1992). The protocol for CAP testing determines if competing noise prevents someone from interpreting or remembering what is heard, if degradation of the speech signal interferes with understanding it, if timing and ordering play a role, and how efficiently one can localize and understand speech signals. Disorders of central auditory processing (Auditory Processing Disorder) may be misdiagnosed as ADD/ADHD because they result in inattentiveness, and the listener cannot focus on or relate to what is being said. Preliminary clinical data indicate that auditory processing problems are common in VCFS (Lightfoot, 2003).

### Scheduling

**Newborn hearing screening:** At birth.

**ABR:** ABR is often used as a newborn screening in infancy. It can also be used as needed to identify possible hearing loss if there is suspicion of a deficit.

**Behavioral audiometry:** Beginning in late infancy or early toddler period, once the child has sufficient muscle tone to sit upright and turn her head to a localize sound stimulus, and continuing into adult life as needed.

**Tympanometry:** From infancy to adult life as needed to identify middle ear fluid.

**Auditory Processing:** From about age 7 years, as needed.

## CARDIOLOGY (PEDIATRIC CARDIOLOGY)

The diagnosis of VCFS is most often made in neonates because of the presence of major heart anomalies such as tetralogy of Fallot, interrupted aortic arch, or truncus arteriosus, and in these cases, the child with VCFS will immediately become connected with a pediatric cardiologist and heart surgeon. However, even in those cases in which congenital heart disease has not been detected by primary care physicians, it is important to have a pediatric cardiology consult and an echocardiogram. There are some heart anomalies that are "silent," meaning that they cannot be detected by auscultation and general physical examination. Such cases are important to identify for a number of reasons, including the need to apply prophylactic antibiotics to protect against bacterial endocarditis during certain medical, surgical, and dental procedures.

## Scheduling

**Cardiology assessment:** If there is an obvious manifestation of heart anomalies, at the earliest possible time after birth or detection. If there are no obvious manifestations of congenital heart disease, an examination should be scheduled as early in life as is practical to rule out silent anomalies.

**Echocardiography:** At the time of initial cardiac assessment.

## CARDIOTHORACIC SURGERY

In most places, the cardiothoracic surgeons work in close synchrony with pediatric cardiologists in order to determine the need for treatment and the timing for it once it has been deemed necessary. The surgeon is usually contacted once a pediatric cardiologist has made a diagnosis of the specific type of congenital heart disease. The management of the heart anomalies in VCFS does not seem to be different from the same anomalies in children who do not have VCFS (Anaclerio et al., 2004). However, postoperative management may be different in relation to issues involving feeding, airway, muscle tone, and risk of infection. The surgeon should therefore be well informed about the special needs of a child with VCFS, such as the potential for hypocalcemia, thrombocytopenia, and immune system dysfunction. In older children and adolescents who sometimes require secondary heart surgery, thrombocytopenia becomes a more pressing concern such that platelet counts should be ordered prior to surgery, and if thrombocytopenia is noted, clotting times should be assessed prior to surgery.

## Scheduling

**Heart surgery:** As indicated based on cardiology assessment.

## CLINICAL GENETICS AND GENETIC COUNSELING

The majority of individuals diagnosed with VCFS today are detected from screenings by pediatric cardiologists when a major conotruncal heart anomaly is detected after birth, or earlier following prenatal detection of these types of heart anomalies. If a fetus is found to have a tetralogy of Fallot, interrupted aortic arch type B, or truncus arteriosus on fetal ultrasound, prenatal screening with FISH for a 22q11.2 deletion is performed. The detection rates for VCFS among fetuses with these heart anomalies is very high. and prenatal detection can help to prepare both parents and physicians for the resulting birth. Parents can be counseled at this time but should also be seen after birth and heart surgery for additional counseling. For cases in which conotruncal heart anomalies are detected after birth, it is the practice in most settings to screen for 22q11.2 deletions. Once the diagnosis is made, counseling should be provided immediately. Often, FISH is not ordered by clinical geneticists, but by other practitioners who have seen the baby first, such as pediatric cardiologists. Unfortunately, in those cases, appropriate counseling may not be provided because the specialist ordering the test may not have expertise in counseling or the time to spend several hours with the family to provide them with needed information and support. In reviewing our cases involving diagnoses by FISH during screening, we have found that fewer than 10% received counseling by a genetic counselor or clinical geneticist.

Although screening of babies with major heart anomalies will detect many cases of VCFS, many others will be missed. In our series of cases at the VCFS International Center at Upstate Medical University referred over the past 10 years (over 700 cases), 57% did not have tetralogy of Fallot, truncus arteriosus, or interrupted aortic arch. Among these cases, the most common anomaly was ventricular septal defect, often in combination with other anomalies such as patent ductus arteriosus, right-sided aortic arch, aortic valve anomalies, or atrial septal defect. In addition, approximately 30% of individuals with VCFS have no congenital heart disease. This means that screening based on the presence of major heart anomalies will miss the majority of cases of VCFS. Therefore, diagnosis is dependent on recognition of a pattern of anomalies that can be highly variable from person to person. This type of expertise typically rests with a clinical geneticist. As a general rule of thumb, any child that has more than one major anomaly, such as the combination of cleft palate with inguinal hernia or developmental delay with unilateral renal agenesis, should be referred to a clinical geneticist.

### Scheduling

**Clinical genetics evaluation:** As soon as possible.

**Cytogenetics and molecular genetics:** At the time of referral to the clinical geneticist.

**Genetic counseling:** After all laboratory tests have been completed and the diagnosis confirmed. For individuals who have VCFS, multiple counseling sessions are often necessary.

## DENTISTRY AND ORTHODONTICS

Children with VCFS have a number of dental problems that may be seen as early as the time of initial dental eruption and last into adult life. The primary dentition (also referred to as deciduous dentition, baby teeth, or milk teeth) is often smaller than normal in VCFS, and the enamel may be deficient or abnormal (Klingberg, Oskarsdottir, Johannesson, & Noren, 2002; Klingberg et al., 2005), resulting in rampant caries and the need for dental restorations or extractions. The secondary dentition (also referred to as succedaneous dentition or permanent teeth) may also have similar anomalies, although the frequency of dental structure problems and rampant caries is far lower. However, once the secondary dentition is in place, malocclusions are commonplace and orthodontic treatment may be needed. It is therefore recommended that a pediatric dentist be consulted by 2 years of age and that the dentist be aware of the problems associated with VCFS that might require more frequent dental scrutiny, such as hypocalcemia, reflux, or dietary preferences. Of course, children with VCFS are also prone to commonplace problems that affect other children, such as milk or juice bottle caries, lack of fluoridation in the local water supply, and a thumb sucking habit. If the child with VCFS also has an immune deficiency or immune disorder, she may be more prone to oral bacterial colonies that could affect the dentition. Children with VCFS also can also develop other oral pathology related to immune disorders, such as thrush and other unusual infections.

Orthodontic issues become evident as the secondary dentition erupts. Facial structure in VCFS, although not grossly abnormal, has a tendency towards vertical maxillary excess, a steep mandibular plane angle, and mild retrognathia (Arvystas & Shprintzen, 1984). Chronic upper airway obstruction from hypertrophic tonsils plus hypotonia can also lead to long-term mouth breathing, which has the additional effect on facial growth of increased facial lengthening. This combination of structural variations results in a face that looks longer than normal, and it can lead to dental arch abnormalities that require maxillary expansion and tooth alignment. Treatment often includes functional appliance therapy. The treatment in VCFS is not different from that required in the general population, but there are specific ramifications of management that need to be coordinated with other therapies. For example, dental appliances, particularly certain types of palatal expanders, can interfere with articulation and hamper some aspects of speech therapy at least temporarily. The presence of metal brackets and dental wires can interfere with magnetic resonance studies that might be required prior to pharyngeal surgery. These types of interactions require someone who will serve as a type of clinical coordinator for the patient.

One aspect of orthodontic evaluation that can be very useful long term is the use of serial cephalometric and panoramic radiographs to plot facial growth. These radiographic studies may be of particular importance in individuals with VCFS who develop juvenile rheumatoid arthritis (JRA) because the mandible in particular can show significant changes with time as a result of JRA. Changes in mandibular shape and position can contribute to compromise of the airway over time. If changes in the shape of the mandibular condyle are observed, referral for evaluation of JRA should be made.

## Scheduling

**Pediatric dentistry:** Prior to 2 years of age.

**Orthodontics:** First evaluation to collect baseline data should be scheduled at approximately 5 or 6 years of age, with therapy often scheduled in the mixed dentition stage, ranging between 7 and 12 years of age.

# DEVELOPMENTAL PEDIATRICS

Developmental pediatricians play an important role in evaluating early developmental delays and recommending specific forms of management that help the child develop and provide the parents with strategies to help their child. The assessments and diagnoses of developmental pediatricians overlap considerably with those of neuropsychologists who specialize in early child development, and both specialists may be called upon when developmental delays are evident. However, development in VCFS tends to be borderline normal or only mildly delayed. Therefore, it is important to have an evaluation by someone familiar with early childhood development who can help to distinguish between those things that are normal and those that clearly require attention.

## Scheduling

**Developmental pediatric assessment:** At the first sign of developmental delay. One year of age or shortly after is a reasonable target age.

# ENDOCRINE EVALUATION

Although routine endocrinological tests can be performed by primary care physicians, most children with VCFS eventually require the attention of an endocrinologist for calcium metabolism, thyroid hormone abnormalities, or parathyroid abnormalities. Examination by an endocrinologist would be most important in infancy if a child had hypocalcemia. Serum calcium and ionized calcium should be checked in all children with VCFS on a regular basis. In older children, routine endocrine tests, such as thyroid function tests, can be performed by primary care physicians, but at any sign of abnormality, a specialist should be consulted. A variety of hormone level tests may be needed to determine if the individual with VCFS has a disorder that could affect performance, mood, or metabolism and potentially cause seizures or life-threatening immune disorders. The most common endocrine disorders in VCFS are hypocalcemia and thyroid problems. Hypocalcemia is often transient and not necessarily a lifelong problem. In some cases, hypocalcemia presents in infancy but then resolves with age. In others, there is no evidence for hypocalcemia early in life but it becomes evident during the teen years. In still others, hypocalcemia may occur intermittently when the person is under stress or is dehydrated or malnourished. For cases in which hypocalcemia is a problem, parathyroid hormone levels should be checked.

Thyroid disorders can include hypothyroidism, hyperthyroidism (Graves' disease), and autoimmune thyroiditis and Hashimoto's disease. Thyroid problems can have a significant effect on mood, and this can be confused with some of the potential psychiatric findings associated with VCFS.

Thymic hormone may also be deficient. Absent thymus has been reported in VCFS, an observation typically based on radiographs taken when heart anomalies are repaired. The fact that the thymus gland is not found does not mean that there is a complete absence of thymus tissue or thymic hormone. Thymus tissue is occasionally scattered in unusual locations in the chest or neck. Only a complete absence of thymic hormone will signal true absence of the thymus or thymic activity, which results in severe immune deficiency.

Endocrinologists also assess patients for growth abnormalities, and key to recommending treatment for growth abnormalities is determining if there is a true growth deficiency as opposed to acquired short stature. In order to determine if short stature is present, serial heights and weights over time are compared to established norms. The standard norms used by most pediatricians in the United States are the data published by the Centers for Disease Control and Prevention (CDC), which are available to anyone at http://www.cdc.gov/growthcharts/. The CDC growth charts are based on normative data collected on thousands of children, adolescents, and adults in order to calculate the mean height, weight, head circumference, body mass index, and weight to height proportion for the general population. The question is if the growth of people with VCFS should be compared to these norms. The short answer is no, and this will be discussed in detail in Chapter 5. The reason is that genetic alterations, especially those involving multiple genes, almost always alter growth patterns, and many syndromes including Down syndrome, achondroplasia, and Williams syndrome have their own growth curves. If it can be demonstrated that children with VCFS do not grow like children who have all of their genes in two copies, then comparing them to the normal growth curves is a mistake that can lead to wrong and potentially dangerous treatment decisions that will alter quality of life in a very significant way. In fact, low weight or reduced linear growth may have nothing to do with nutrition in many if not nearly all children with VCFS.

### Schedule

**Endocrine evaluation:** Endocrine evaluations can be scheduled at any time beginning in infancy and are usually recommended based on symptoms. These would include hypocalcemia, hypothyroidism, hypoparathyroidism, hypopituitarism, delayed bone age, or severe short stature.

## GASTROENTEROLOGY (PEDIATRIC GASTROENTEROLOGY)

The challenge in children with VCFS is to determine if feeding problems are due to swallowing difficulty, airway compromise, or problems associated with the eating process or if a perceived problem is not actually a problem at all. As will be discussed in the next chapter, weight gain and growth are easily misinterpreted in VCFS if those making judgments are unfamiliar with the syndrome. Children with any kind of eating problem are typically diagnosed with dysphagia or swallowing problems. However, feeding issues in VCFS are very complex and require careful diagnostic expertise to decipher. Gastroenterology deals with problems from the esophagus through the rest of the digestive tract. Children with VCFS can have esophageal problems that are associated with compression by anomalous major vessels in the chest, such as aberrant subclavian arteries and vascular rings. Some patients, particularly those with more severe hypotonia, have GER or GERD, and this can cause esophageal erosions. On occasion, GER and GERD are actually induced by overfeeding in an attempt to promote weight gain. Gastric problems may present as persistent emesis (often misinterpreted as reflux), often related to slow gastric emptying accompanied by overfeeding. Intestinal problems are commonly related to slow motility of the gut resulting in chronic constipation. Therefore, patients with VCFS often need to see a gastroenterologist, but it is important for that specialist to understand the special nature of VCFS and the many possible layers of problems that cover every portion of the digestive tract. First referral often comes in infancy because of emesis, reflux, or chronic constipation (all of which may occur in combination).

## Schedule

**Gastroenterology assessment:** Depending on age of presentation of feeding problem or constipation.

# IMMUNOLOGY EVALUATION

Although immunologic deficiency is a key diagnostic feature of the DiGeorge sequence, as discussed in Chapter 2, severe immune deficiency is not a common feature in VCFS. However, immune disorders with chronic respiratory infections, middle ear disease, and urinary tract infections are common. It is important to treat these issues properly without making assumptions about the cause of either the illness or the response to the illness. Excessive treatment with antibiotics can lead to opportunistic infections by more unusual microbes, including fungi and exotic bacteria. Therefore, input from a specialist in immune function or infectious diseases is indicated. If a child with VCFS has recurring bronchitis or pneumonia, then it is especially important to have this assessment done. Laboratory tests to identify specific risk factors, safety for giving live virus vaccines, and the need for special forms of treatment including intravenous immunoglobulin (IVIG) should be done when there is evidence for a severe immune disorder.

The immune evaluation in the first year of life would include physical examination and a panel of laboratory tests that should be completed before giving live virus vaccines. Live virus vaccines include measles, mumps, rubella, and varicella. The Sabin oral polio vaccine is also a live but attenuated virus vaccine, while the Salk vaccine is an inactivated virus vaccine. In rare cases, the Sabin vaccine can cause polio-related symptoms if B-lymphocyte activity is abnormal. Testing in infants varies according to age and clinical history, including the history of immunizations. Infants should receive a complete blood count with differential and platelets, an assessment of the total numbers of antibodies or immunoglobulins in the blood, and analysis of T-lymphocytes (lymphocyte subsets). Low counts of T-lymphocyte subsets known as CD4 (helper cells) and CD8 cells signal an immune deficiency. People with immune deficiencies contract disease more often and also contract a larger variety of viral and bacterial illnesses, including uncommon opportunistic infections. The presence of thrush or other fungal infections or unusual bacterial infections should be a source of concern and close follow-up with an immunologist. In many cases of VCFS, the number of lymphocytes may be low, but the function of these cells is normal. In these cases, there is no increased risk for severe immunodeficiency that would lead to rare and opportunistic infections, and live viral vaccines can usually be given. If lymphocyte function is abnormal, even if the count is normal, live viral vaccines should not be given. Influenza vaccine is a different story. All children with VCFS should receive flu vaccines annually at the recommended ages. Flu vaccines are not live virus vaccines. It is also recommended that everyone in close contact with children who have VCFS receive the flu vaccine. Treatment with intravenous antibodies may be necessary in cases of severe immune deficiency.

In most people with VCFS, immune function improves over time, but if problems persist, a formal immune system evaluation should be performed at the first opportunity. It is also important that primary care physicians and others not overreact to frequent respiratory illnesses or overinterpret chronic congestion. We often encounter cases in which the presence of green mucus in the upper respiratory tract is interpreted as a severe bacterial infection or something more than what it truly is, a simple chemical reaction in the body. Green secretion color is caused by a chemical reaction in the body to any infecting virus or bacteria. White blood cells cluster to defend the body from the pathogen, and the chemical reaction produces a substance similar to chlorine that turns the mucus green. In many instances, antibiotics are prescribed without cultures confirming a bacterial infection. The unnecessary use of antibiotics if the infection is viral rather than bacterial can cause illness by killing bacteria that normally inhabit the respiratory tract and allowing antibiotic-resistant strains to take their place. Treatment may result in making children medically dependent.

## Schedule

**Immunologic evaluation:**  First year of life and as needed following.

## MAGNETIC RESONANCE IMAGING AND ANGIOGRAPHY

Individuals with VCFS have been reported to have variations in brain anatomy including reduced cerebral volumes, small cerebellum, reduced volume of the corpus callosum, frequent cavum septum pellucidum, white matter hyperintensities, and cystic structures. These variations have not been shown to have any specific predictive power relative to cognitive performance or the development of mental illness to date. However, there are a number of findings that have significant implications for cognitive development including polymicrogyria and pachygyria (Ehara, Maegaki, & Takeshita, 2003; Koolen et al., 2004; Robin et al., 2006) and cortical dysgenesis (Bird, 2001; Bird & Scambler, 2000). In cases of severe developmental delay, MR scans of the brain are indicated. Although there are no treatments for severe brain anomalies, the information may dramatically alter counseling with regard to prognosis.

In patients with seizures that are clearly not related to hypocalcemia, MR imaging of the brain will be needed to see if the seizures are secondary to strokes or other brain anomalies. Strokes occasionally occur in individuals with VCFS either secondary to heart surgery that can result in thromboses and an embolism in the brain (a risk of heart surgery in general), or because of vascular anomalies that result in a blockage of a blood vessel.

Magnetic resonance angiography (MRA) to locate the internal carotid arteries has been recommended for all patients with VCFS undergoing pharyngeal flap surgery (Mitnick, Bello, Golding-Kushner, Argamaso, & Shprintzen, 1996; Tatum, Chang, Havkin, & Shprintzen, 2002). One paper argued against the need for preoperative MRA because of the additional cost to the medical system, using a small series of cases and limited questionnaire evidence from a small sample of surgeons as justification for their conclusion (Witt, Miller, Marsh, Muntz, & Grames, 1998). The article was followed by a discussion and rejection of the data presented based on the very small sample size and failure to demonstrate sufficient evidence to refute the potential risk that was subsequently reported by Tatum et al. (2002). MRA is not necessary for tonsillectomy or adenoidectomy because incisions are not made in the posterior pharyngeal wall and the internal carotids are not in the operative field.

In cases where there is sufficient permanent metal in the body of a patient with VCFS, it may be necessary to substitute CT angiography or CT scans for MR because magnetic metals such as stainless steel degrade the MR image and pose potential risks to the patient because of the very strong magnet in the MR scanner. In some cases, small amounts of metal that are not in the visual field may not hamper the examination.

## Scheduling

**MR imaging of the brain (MRI):** When required to identify an abnormality.

**MR angiography (MRA):** Immediately prior to pharyngeal flap or pharyngoplasties, which should not be done prior to 4 years of age in the majority of cases

## NASOPHARYNGOSCOPY, FEES OR FEESST, DIRECT LARYNGOSCOPY, BRONCHOSCOPY, ESOPHAGOSCOPY, AND GASTROSCOPY

Endoscopic procedures are often used to directly visualize the anatomy of the upper airway or digestive tract. Fiberoptic endoscopy of the upper airway is important for assessing a number of concerns in VCFS, including upper airway patency, velopharyngeal function, vocal cord function, swallowing (FEES or FEESST), and anatomy of the palate, pharynx, and larynx. Although the technical aspects of endoscopy can be applied at any time, nasopharyngoscopy for the purposes of assessing speech are extremely difficult to apply in children under the age of 4 years because of a lack of compliance resulting in the inability to obtain a usable speech sample. Because the information obtained from this procedure is so critical to surgical success, the procedure should not be scheduled for speech purposes before there is sufficient speech development to obtain a varied speech sample.

There are other circumstances, however, that demand upper airway fiberoptic endoscopy prior to 4 years of age to obtain information critical to management of difficult problems in infants and toddlers. Airway compromise is common in VCFS as discussed in Chapter 2. Robin sequence, hypotonia, tonsillar hypertrophy, laryngeal web, laryngomalacia, or laryngeal paralysis can all lead to airway problems that are best diagnosed using fiberoptic endoscopy with the patient awake. Nasopharyngoscopy should be completely painless when done properly and there should be no reason to defer the examination. The procedure can be applied as early as the neonatal period.

Another commonly applied fiberoptic technique is the evaluation of swallowing with FEES or FEESST. FEES is an acronym for Fiberoptic Endoscopic Evaluation of Swallowing and FEESST adds Sensory Testing to the protocol. The purpose of FEES and FEESST is to rule out aspiration while being able to determine if there are normal movements of the vocal cords, arytenoids, epiglottis, and upper esophageal sphincter using a variety of food stimuli. It has been found that radiation exposure to the neck significantly increases the risk of thyroid cancer in adult life (Hall & Holm, 1998) and that exposure of the brain to diagnostic doses of radiation in infants can also have a deleterious effect on brain growth and function (Hall et al., 2004). This is a major advantage of FEES and FEESST over videofluoroscopic swallowing studies. FEES and FEESST can be performed at any age depending on the need for instrumental assessment of swallowing. In most cases, a careful clinical assessment of swallowing is sufficient to rule out aspiration or serious swallowing problems, and instrumental procedures are probably necessary in less than 10% of all cases. In those cases, FEES should be the frontline procedure in order to limit radiation exposure to the thyroid gland. These examinations would be ordered based on symptomatic presentation.

Direct laryngoscopy to assess laryngeal anatomy can actually be a part of a fiberoptic assessment of the upper airway or nasopharyngoscopy for speech evaluation. Abnormal respiratory sounds such as stridor or stertor often signal the need to assess the larynx because of the rather high prevalence of laryngeal anomalies in VCFS. Laryngomalacia in particular is very common (see Video 2–10), but the symptoms and presentation of this relatively benign condition can overlap with the presentation of laryngeal web (see Figure 2–50), and direct visualization should therefore be performed. Membranous laryngeal webs are often easy to treat when necessary, so early identification is important. Once the web is seen, direct laryngoscopy under anesthesia is typically scheduled. Bronchoscopy should be performed at the same time because of the high prevalence of vascular anomalies that could compress the trachea.

GI endoscopy procedures (esophagoscopy and gastroscopy) are also indicated in some cases of VCFS that present with persistent emesis or symptoms consistent with gastroesophageal reflux. Unfortunately, the term *reflux* has become associated with a variety of digestive tract issues that include emesis (including nasal regurgitation), spitting up, and limited food intake. True gastroesophageal reflux implies that food has reached the stomach and that stomach contents, typically gastric acid with or without food mixed in, escape the lower esophageal sphincter and enter the esophagus causing discomfort, heartburn, pain, and occasionally some extraesophageal escape of a small amount of vomitus. Emesis should not be confused with reflux because the conditions might be different, as discussed in Chapter 2 in detail. Diagnostic procedures for confirming true GER and GERD would include pH probes and esophagoscopy, which can document tissue changes in the esophageal mucosa. Esophagoscopy can also show vascular compressions that might cause a stricture or a diverticulum. These procedures would also be ordered as symptoms present, and this could be at any point after birth.

## Schedule

**Nasopharyngoscopy (for speech):** Four years of age or later, if speech is hypernasal or hyponasal or if voice is hoarse.

**Nasopharyngoscopy (for airway assessment):** When needed based on symptom presentation.

**FEES or FEESST:** When needed based on symptom presentation.

**Direct laryngoscopy, bronchoscopy:** When needed based on symptom presentation.

**Esophagoscopy and gastroscopy:** When needed based on symptom presentation.

## NEPHROLOGY

Renal anomalies and genitourinary problems are not among the most common of anomalies, but they do occur frequently enough that a nephrologist should be available for consultation. This includes electrolyte abnormalities and blood pressure anomalies that can be related to calcium, sodium, and other electrolyte metabolism. These problems are not age dependent in VCFS, but first presentation is often in infancy or early childhood.

## Schedule

**Nephrology evaluation:** When needed based on symptom presentation.

## NEUROLOGY

Seizures are common in VCFS. Once hypocalcemia has been ruled out as a cause of seizures, a neurologist should be consulted to assess these neurologic events and manage treatment. Seizures are not age dependent in VCFS and may occur for the first time in infancy, childhood, late adolescence, or adulthood. Electroencephalography is required to determine the nature of the seizure activity and is ordered by the neurologist when indicated. There is also some overlap of expertise between pediatric neurologists, developmental pediatricians, and child psychiatrists in relation to components of VCFS such as developmental delay, autism spectrum disorder, and ADD/ADHD. Because not every location has all of these specialists available, each specialist should be queried regarding level of comfort in dealing with these symptom complexes.

### Schedule

**Neurology evaluation:** As early as possible when symptoms present.

## NEUROPSYCHOLOGY

A neuropsychologist is a specialist who blends expertise in psychology and neuroscience in order to understand how human cognition and behavior are related to neuroanatomy and brain function. Because VCFS is so complex a disorder in relation to brain-related disorders, it is important to have a closely coordinated effort between developmental specialists, neuropsychologists, and psychiatrists so that the interaction between cognitive and psychiatric symptoms can be appreciated. Neuropsychologists perform a variety of age-appropriate tests that are age appropriate to ascertain behavioral disorders at each stage of life and to see if there is a progressive development of symptoms.

### Schedule

**Neuropsychological evaluation:** Beginning at age 2 and periodically into adult life.

## NEUROSURGICAL EVALUATION

A number of anomalies associated with VCFS would prompt referral to a neurosurgeon, including Arnold-Chiari anomaly, syrinx, tethered cord, scoliosis, and on rare occasion, brain anomalies such as hydrocephalus and porencephalic cysts. These problems are not among the most common seen in VCFS and are sometimes detected serendipitously during examinations for other problems. Referral to a neurosurgeon is scheduled when these problems are noted and/or symptomatic.

### Schedule

**Neurosurgical consult:** When needed based on symptom presentation.

## NUTRITION

Nutritional consultations present a tricky situation in children with VCFS. Early feeding can often be fraught with anxiety and tension. Parents sometimes feel guilty because they have a difficult time getting their children to eat. The reasons for feeding difficulty are often misunderstood, as described earlier in Chapter 2. Parents sometimes feel the need to give their children as many calories as they can because they have been told that their children are underweight. Parents may indulge their children with snacks that have poor nutritional value but a lot of calories in an effort to push calories. Nutritionists may recommend better and more nutritious diets, and when these are implemented, children with VCFS who are resistant to change and have the urge to eat sweets may, as might any child, react negatively to the change. It is therefore important to have the nutritionist involved early on with the speech pathologist who is implementing feeding recommendations. Working together, these two specialists can arrange appropriate protocols and, when necessary for transitioning gradually from a "junk" diet to a nutritious one, use principles of behavior modification and sound dietary content.

### Scheduling

**Nutrition consult:** If there are feeding difficulties early in life, the nutritionist should be consulted as early as possible to coordinate a sound diet with feeding therapy implemented by the feeding therapist.

## OPHTHALMOLOGY (PEDIATRIC OPHTHALMOLOGY)

Eye anomalies are common in VCFS. Some are incidental findings that do not require treatment, such as prominent corneal nerves, posterior embryotoxon, and tortuous retinal vessels. However, anomalies such as strabismus do require early detection and treatment in order to prevent amblyopia, a condition that can result in loss of vision in one eye. If an eye muscle imbalance is suspected, the child should be referred immediately for evaluation and treatment that can range from patching one eye to corrective lenses or surgery. Other eye conditions require immediate diagnosis, although treatment is not an issue. The presence of a coloboma, or cleft in the iris, should be assessed to see if the retina and optic nerve are involved; this has implications for vision and underlying brain anatomy. Eye anomalies should be evaluated by an ophthalmologist (who is a medical doctor) rather than an optometrist, who does not have the ability to dilate the eyes and fully assess eye anatomy or treat the problems medically or surgically. However, many ophthalmologists have optometrists in the office to assist with vision testing.

### Schedule

**Ophthalmology (pediatric ophthalmology):** If anomalies or problems are obvious, such as strabismus or coloboma, evaluation should be performed in infancy. All children should have ophthalmic assessment by 2 years of age.

## ORTHOPEDICS

Skeletal anomalies and abnormal muscle stretching in relation to hypotonia can cause leg pains and other orthopedic symptoms that require evaluation. Spinal fusions, scoliosis, and skeletal anomalies are probably underdetected in children with VCFS and can affect multiple areas of the body including the spine, ankles, hands, and feet. Hand problems can range from contractures to extra digits and fused phalanges. Orthopedic consults are scheduled when there is a symptomatic presentation. The majority of VCFS referrals to orthopedists relate to leg pains and gait issues. These problems are sometimes evaluated by podiatrists and physical therapists and, if there are no structural anomalies of the skeleton, it is possible that any or all of these specialists may treat leg pains appropriately.

### Schedule

**Orthopedic evaluation:** When needed based on symptom presentation.

## OTOLARYNGOLOGY

An otolaryngologist is involved in the care of nearly all children with VCFS because of respiratory problems, middle ear disease, voice problems, resonance disorders and velopharyngeal insufficiency. The frequent need for tonsillectomy, myringotomy and tubes, laryngoscopy and bronchoscopy, and nasopharyngoscopy typically means that otolaryngologists are involved in the care of a child with VCFS beginning early in life, often in the neonatal period. Symptoms that should prompt referral to an otolaryngologist include stridor or stertor in infancy, multiple middle ear infections in 1 year, hearing loss, sleep disordered breathing, chronic cough or choking, hoarseness, and velopharyngeal insufficiency.

### Schedule

**Otolaryngology consult:** If upper airway obstruction, stridor, or stertor are present in the neonatal period, assessment should be scheduled immediately. Otherwise, consult is arranged when needed based on symptom presentation of airway, voice, hearing, or other relevant problems.

## PHYSICAL THERAPY

The primary problem that prompts referral to a physical therapist in children with VCFS is the complaint of chronic leg pain. Leg pains in VCFS are most often the result of pronation with resulting abnormal stretching of the leg muscles. The physical therapist can prescribe and implement appropriate muscle stretching and relaxation techniques to prevent these pains. It is also appropriate for physical therapists to teach the parents of affected children the necessary stretching routines so they can be implemented on a daily basis at home.

### Schedule

**Physical therapy:** Early childhood evaluation for tightening of the heel cords and other lower limb anomalies.

## PODIATRY

Leg pains are often related to flat foot arches that cause abnormal stretching on the muscles of the legs, resulting in pains in the calves and shins and sometimes the knees and thighs. These findings were initially reported at an annual meeting of the VCFS Educational Foundation, Inc. by Dr. Ahmad Al-Khattat and colleagues from Northampton, Great Britain. Dr. Al-Khattat reported his data on leg pains in VCFS at several international meetings, and that information is posted on the Web site of the Velo-Cardio-Facial Syndrome Educational Foundation, Inc., (www.vcfsef.org), at the specific URL of http://www.vcfsef. org/pp/3YearProspectiveStudy/index.htm. These types of leg pains can often be treated successfully with soft insoles to gently raise the instep and prevent pronation.

## Schedule

**Podiatric assessment:** There is merit to early examination of all individuals with VCFS to determine if there is sufficient severity of pronation to warrant the use of soft insoles. This assessment could be done by a podiatrist, physical therapist, or orthopedist. The treatment typically consists of appropriate stretching exercises to be administered at home.

# PSYCHIATRY

Psychiatric problems (inclusive of psychosis, but not restricted to psychosis) are common in VCFS and may be the most difficult to face for parents. Although it is clear that psychiatric issues are directly linked to the deletion, thus squarely placing the cause with genomics rather than parenting, there is still a stigma associated with mental illness and parents may feel responsible. The majority of referrals of adolescent and adult patients to the VCFS International Center in Syracuse have not seen a psychiatrist. It is typically only the most severely mentally ill patients who reach the center with a history of treatment by a psychiatrist. Parents of younger patients or those with less severe mental illness have tended to indicate that early treatments have been prescribed by pediatricians or family practice physicians rather than by child psychiatrists. The most common early psychiatric diagnosis in children with VCFS is ADD/ADHD. Other common diagnoses also include obsessive-compulsive disorder, oppositional-defiant disorder, and impulsivity. Although early psychosis that would demand referral to a psychiatrist is not common, the early manifestations of behavioral problems should instigate such a referral. In a way, the situation is analogous to waiting to see a dentist until an abscess has occurred instead of taking care of a cavity in its earliest presentation. We recommend seeing a child psychiatrist in childhood, no later than school age. Although not all children with VCFS will require treatment (in fact, it may be a minority of cases at that stage), it is important to have behavior analyzed by a professional who specializes in this area. There is also tremendous value in having both a neuropsychologist and a psychiatrist performing evaluations at about the same time because problems of cognition and mental functioning may be interrelated.

## Schedule

**Psychiatric assessment:** School age.

# PULMONOLOGY (PEDIATRIC PULMONOLOGY)

Problems associated with the lower airway and lungs require the input of a pulmonologist, especially in infancy and childhood. Recurrent pneumonias, asthma, reactive airway disease, and structural anomalies that can impair the function of the lungs require proper assessment and treatment. Respiration is also closely connected to circulation, so children with pulmonary valve and artery anomalies also require pulmonary assessment. Pulmonary function tests should be performed to assess lung capacity. However, the pulmonologist should be aware of how velopharyngeal insufficiency might affect the outcome of pulmonary function tests because of the potential for loss of air through the nasal cavity during hard blowing for the test. The use of noseclips during the study may not necessarily completely impede the flow of air through the nose and could result in a false positive for diminished lung capacity.

## Schedule

**Pulmonary assessment:** As early as possible if there is a history of pulmonary valve or artery problems, chronic lower respiratory illness, and a history consistent with asthma or reactive airway disease.

# RECONSTRUCTIVE SURGERY

The primary need for reconstructive surgery in children with VCFS is for speech purposes. Cleft palate repair is necessary for those children born with overt clefts of the palate, and for those who have velopharyngeal insufficiency, pharyngeal flap surgery is an option after 4 years of age. This type of reconstructive surgery is done by a number of different specialists depending on location, training, and experience. Otolaryngologists (most often facial plastic surgeons, but occasionally pediatric otolaryngologists), plastic surgeons, some pediatric surgeons, and some oral-maxillofacial surgeons perform these operations. If overt cleft palate is involved, most surgeons prefer to repair these clefts at or before 1 year of age. We do not recommend surgical repair of submucous cleft palate because these procedures are rarely successful in children with VCFS in terms of resolving velopharyngeal insufficiency. It is preferred to treat their velopharyngeal insufficiency with pharyngeal flap after 4 years of age in order to obtain accurate diagnostic information that will improve the surgical outcome while reducing complications (Shprintzen et al., 1979; Shprintzen, Singer, Sidoti, & Argamaso, 1992; Tatum, Chang, Havkin, & Shprintzen, 2002).

In some cases, there may be a desire to perform reconstructive surgery on the nose or jaws of someone with VCFS for either functional or esthetic reasons. Rhinoplasties (often called "nose jobs") are done by both otolaryngologists (facial plastic surgeons) and plastic surgeons. Jaw surgery is also done by these specialists and by oral-maxillofacial surgeons. Jaw surgery is not typically recommended before late teen years when growth is complete. The one exception is babies with Robin sequence, in which case distraction of the lower jaw may be recommended in the neonatal period.

### Schedule

**Reconstructive surgery:** In infancy if there is overt cleft palate or Robin sequence; 4 years of age if velopharyngeal insufficiency requires surgical reconstruction. Rhinoplasty and jaw reconstruction during late teen years if desired.

## RENAL ULTRASOUND

Small kidneys, unilateral absence of a kidney, cystic kidneys, hydronephrosis, and vesicoureteral reflux are all features of VCFS and happen commonly enough to warrant renal ultrasound.

### Schedule

**Renal ultrasound:** When the diagnosis of VCFS is made.

## SPEECH-LANGUAGE EVALUATION

A common misconception is that one cannot have a speech-language evaluation if the patient is not talking. This would be like saying that if your automobile's engine will not start, there is no reason to bring the car to a mechanic. With rare exception, children with VCFS develop speech. The majority of them have velopharyngeal insufficiency, and of those, most will have severe velopharyngeal insufficiency. Moreover, of those, most develop severe compensatory articulation disorders. In addition, many of these children have significant delays in expressive language. It is a good idea to begin speech-language consults with parents prior to the onset of speech to teach parents how to recognize abnormal patterns of articulation that might develop and how to treat them at home so that they will not continue to appear in the child's early vocalizations. The speech pathologist who understands VCFS (and speech and language development in general) will be able to teach the parent skills designed to stimulate the child's use of speech and how to produce speech sounds. The general principles of this process will be described in detail in the second volume of this series on VCFS.

## Schedule

**Feeding evaluation:** As soon as problem is identified.

**Speech-language evaluation:** Prior to first birthday.

**Speech therapy:** As soon as need is identified.

# UROLOGY

Urologic anomalies occur relatively infrequently in VCFS, but males with VCFS have hypospadias, cryptorchidism, and inguinal hernias at a rate higher than seen in the general population. Occasional urethral anomalies may also be encountered, but rarely. All of these anomalies are surgically correctable, and referral to a urologist should be made in the first year of life to determine the ideal timing for these operations.

## Schedule

**Urological assessment:** In infancy.

# VIDEOFLUOROSCOPY FOR SPEECH

Although many centers rely on nasopharyngoscopy alone to assess velopharyngeal function, videofluoroscopy in lateral and frontal views is essential to the accurate diagnosis of movements in the velopharyngeal valve (Golding-

Kushner et al., 1990). Because ionizing radiation is involved, the procedure is not scheduled until it is certain that the patient will have reconstructive surgery for velopharyngeal insufficiency, and it is critical that the patient be compliant and have sufficient language development to provide a varied speech sample for the study. We therefore typically schedule these studies to assess velopharyngeal function during speech at 4 years of age or later. This provides sufficient time to apply treatment before school age so that the affected individual enters school with normal speech.

## Schedule

**Multiview videofluoroscopy:** Four years of age or after.

## VIDEOFLUOROSCOPY FOR SWALLOWING

Videofluoroscopy to assess swallowing is referred to as MBSS, or modified barium swallow study, if different food stimuli are presented during the study. If only liquid barium is used, the study is simply referred to as a barium swallow study. Many clinicians regard the MBSS as the gold standard for swallowing or feeding problems. However, we do not. A clinician with expertise in this area who performs careful clinical evaluation of swallowing that includes cervical auscultation is able to assess disorders of the oral stage and most aspects of the actual swallow. We prefer to use FEES if an instrumental technique is necessary to rule out aspiration. Aspiration is actually quite rare in VCFS (and in children in general), although pneumonia is common because of immune disorder. Our experience is that instrumental studies have been necessary in fewer than 10% of our referrals, and of those, only several cases of true aspiration have been found. MBSS studies provide direct radiation to the thyroid gland. This type of radiation exposure is especially dangerous to the thyroid gland in infants and toddlers and should be avoided unless there is no other option. We have not performed a MBSS study in a patient with VCFS in more than 10 years. Simple, brief barium swallows are sometimes required to determine if there is an esophageal constriction that might be related to a vascular ring or other vascular anomaly.

## Schedule

**Modified barium swallow:** To be avoided, especially in infancy and early childhood, unless there is no alternative.

# REFERENCES

Anaclerio, S., Di Ciommo, V., Michielon, G., Digilio, M. C., Formigari, R., Picchio, F. M., et al. (2004). Conotruncal heart defects: Impact of genetic syndromes on immediate operative mortality. *Italian Heart Journal*, *5*, 624–628.

Arvystas, M., & Shprintzen, R. J. (1984). Craniofacial morphology in the velo-cardio-facial syndrome. *Journal of Craniofacial Genetics and Developmental Biology*, *4*, 39–45.

Bird, L. M. (2001). Cortical dysgenesis and 22q11 deletion. *Clinical Dysmorphology*, *10*, 77.

Bird, L. M., & Scambler, P. (2000). Cortical dysgenesis in 2 patients with chromosome 22q11 deletion. *Clinical Genetics*, *58*, 64–68.

Cutler-Landsman, D. (2007). Educating Children with Velo-Cardio-Facial Syndrome. San Diego: Plural Publishing.

Ehara, H., Maegaki, Y., & Takeshita, K. (2003). Pachygyria and polymicrogyria in 22q11 deletion syndrome. *American Journal of Medical Genetics A*, *117*, 80–82.

Golding-Kushner, K. J., Argamaso, R. V., Cotton, R. T., Grames, L. M., Henningsson, G., Jones, D. L., et al. (1990). Standardization for the reporting of nasopharyngoscopy and multi-view videofluoroscopy: A report from an international working group. *Cleft Palate Journal*, *27*, 337–347.

Hall, P., Adami, H. O., Trichopoulos, D., Pedersen, N. L., Lagiou, P., Ekbom, A., et al. (2004). Effect of low doses of ionising radiation in infancy on cognitive function in adulthood: Swedish population based cohort study. *British Medical Journal*, *3*, *328*(7430), 19.

Hall, P., & Holm, L. E. (1998). Radiation-associated thyroid cancer—Facts and fiction. *Acta Oncologica*, *37*, 325–330.

Katz, J. (1992). Classification of central auditory processing disorders. In J. Katz, N. Stecker, & D. Henderson (Eds.), *Central auditory processing: A transdisciplinary view* (pp. 81–91). St. Louis, MO: Mosby.

Klingberg, G., Dietz, W., Oskarsdottir, S., Odelius, H., Gelander, L., & Noren, J. G. (2005). Morphological appearance and chemical composition of enamel in primary teeth from patients with 22q11 deletion syndrome. *European Journal of Oral Science*, *113*, 303–311.

Klingberg, G., Oskarsdottir, S., Johannesson, E. L., & Noren, J. G. (2002). Oral manifestations in 22q11 deletion syndrome. *International Journal of Paediatric Dentistry*, *12*, 14–23.

Koolen, D. A., Veltman, J. A., Renier, W. O., Droog, R. P., van Kessel, A. G., & de Vries, B. B. A. (2004). Chromosome 22q11 deletion and pachygyria characterized by array-based comparative genomic hybridization. *American Journal of Medical Genetics*, *131A*, 322–324.

Lightfoot, D. (2003, August). *Central auditory processing*. Paper presented at the Ninth Annual International Scientific Meeting of the Velo-Cardio-Facial Syndrome Educational Foundation, Inc., San Diego, CA.

Mitnick, R. J., Bello, J. A., Golding-Kushner, K. J., Argamaso, R. V., & Shprintzen, R. J. (1996). The use of magnetic resonance angiography prior to pharyngeal flap surgery in patients with velo-cardio-facial syndrome. *Plastic and Reconstructive Surgery*, *97*, 908–919.

Robin, N. H., Taylor, C. J., McDonald-McGinn, D. M., Zackai, E. H., Bingham, P., Collins, K. J., et al. (2006). Polymicrogyria and deletion 22q11.2 syndrome: Window to the etiology of a common cortical malformation. *American Journal of Medical Genetics A*, *140*, 2416–2425.

Shprintzen, R. J. (1997). *Genetics, syndromes and communication disorders*. San Diego, CA: Singular.

Shprintzen, R. J. (1998). Discussion of limited value of preoperative cervical vascular imaging in patients with velocardiofacial syndrome. *Plastic and Reconstructive Surgery*, *101*, 1196–1199.

Shprintzen, R. J., Lewin, M. L., Croft, C. B., Daniller, A. I., Argamaso, R. V., Ship, A., et al. (1979). A comprehensive study of pharyngeal flap surgery: tailor-made flaps. *Cleft Palate Journal*, 16, 46–55.

Shprintzen, R. J., Singer, L., Sidoti, E. J., & Argamaso, R. V. (1992). Pharyngeal flap surgery: postoperative complications. *International Anesthesiology Clinics*, *30*, 115–124.

Tatum, S. A., III, Chang, J., Havkin, N., Shprintzen, R. J., (2002). Pharyngeal flap and the internal carotid in velo-cardio-facial syndrome. *Archives of Facial and Plastic Surgery*, *4*, 73–80.

Witt, P. D., Miller, D., Marsh, J. L., Muntz, H. R., & Grames, L. M. (1998). Limited value of preoperative cervical vascular imaging in patients with velocardiofacial syndrome. *Plastic Reconstructive Surgery*, *101*, 1184–1195.

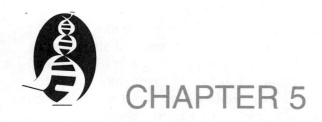

# CHAPTER 5

# Growth, Weight Gain, and Feeding

## BY ROBERT J. SHPRINTZEN, ANNE MARIE HIGGINS, AND ABRAHAM LIPTON

*T*he problems presented by children with VCFS can be numerous and may seem overwhelming, especially for new parents. Part of our job as health care professionals is to avoid complicating life even more. Stated differently, we must adhere to the Hippocratic oath and "do no harm." Our experience of more than 30 years with VCFS (60 years combined) has shown us that one of the areas most fraught with the potential for making children medically dependent and hurting their quality of life and that of the entire family is early feeding difficulties. There are issues related to feeding difficulties and weight gain in VCFS that are often overlooked. To address these issues, it became clear that we needed to understand more about physical growth and development in VCFS.

## IS SHORT STATURE A FEATURE OF VCFS?

In the earliest reports of VCFS, we described "relative short statue" as a clinical finding. Most of the children described in the 1978 paper had height and weight in the normal range, but all were below the 25th centile for both measures. Two children in the sample were below the 3rd centile for height and weight. In subsequent studies, the frequency of reported short stature increased (Motzkin, Marion, Goldberg, Shprintzen, & Saenger, 1993; Young, Shprintzen, & Goldberg, 1980), ranging up to 50% of cases studied. All data reported in these early studies were cross-sectional and very few adults with VCFS were encountered, so it was not possible to determine how many eventually reached normal heights.

Because we have been able to follow most of our patients from the earlier studies into adulthood, we have had the opportunity to see that none of those cases we followed early in life were of very short stature. In fact, all were within the normal range of height. In many cases, we were able to determine that they had reached "expected height," meaning the height one would expect based on parental height as calculated by percentile. We also had the opportunity to determine that none of our patients had been treated with growth hormone to enhance their height.

It also occurred to us that people with other multiple anomaly syndromes, such as Down syndrome or Williams syndrome, are known to grow differently than the general population. Therefore, comparing them to norms established for the general population, such as those published by the CDC, is not done. Individuals with Down syndrome, Williams syndrome, achondroplasia, and other multiple anomaly syndromes have their own growth curves that provide normative data for people with those specific disorders. Why then would we expect that people with VCFS who are missing 40 genes from one copy of chromosome 22 would grow like people who have those 40 genes? Might there be a growth curve for VCFS that differs from the general population? Would a different growth velocity for VCFS mean that comparing height and weight to the CDC norms for the general population is a mistake that could lead to erroneous treatment decisions?

In order to construct a growth curve for VCFS, we maximized the amount of data we would obtain by using longitudinal data collected on the hundreds of patients we have followed over the past 30 years. However, we also wanted to utilize individual measurements by including patients we have followed for shorter periods of time but for whom we had at least two measurements more than 1 year apart. We had data on a total of 1085 individuals, with a total of 8196 data points among them for height and 10,237 data points for weight. In addition, we had birth weight data for all cases from parental recollection and/or medical records. We found parental recollection of birth weights to be very accurate. Data were available into adulthood for 196 cases. Males and females were nearly equally represented in the samples, with 556 males and 529 females.

All data points (height and weight) were recorded to the nearest month of age and segregated according to sex. We were concerned that congenital heart disease (CHD) might play a role in eventual growth outcomes, so we then separated those cases with heart disease from those without. The presence or absence of heart disease was determined by review of medical records in combination with parental report and examination by our team in the majority of cases. Not all cases had echocardiography, especially the older cases, but cases seen within the past decade did. Some of the oldest cases had cardiac catheterization to confirm specific heart lesions, and operative histories were reviewed. Of the total sample, 758 (just under 70%) had histories of CHD. The number of data points for the heart disease group was 5922, with 2315 for the non–heart disease group. Among those with heart disease, we culled out those cases with pulmonary stenosis or atresia, hypothesizing that they would be most prone to growth problems because of poor peripheral perfusion. Only 6% of the total sample, 65 cases, had pulmonary atresia or stenosis.

For each month of age, mean weight and height were calculated, and standard deviations were also calculated. There were sufficient numbers for all ages between birth and 16 years of age for these calculations to be meaningful. There were smaller numbers of subjects beyond 16 years of age with fewer data points. Therefore, data were pooled in 4-month intervals to have sufficient numbers to calculate meaningful means and standard deviations.

We also looked at expected heights for our adult patients for those who were able to provide us with paternal and maternal data. We were able to do this for 127 cases (60 males, 67 females). Expected heights were calculated using the formulae:

For males:  (paternal height + maternal height + 5) / 2

For females:  (paternal height + maternal height − 5) / 2

These formulae have been found to have approximately 90% accuracy in the general population.

The growth curves for the total data including all cases are shown in Figure 5–1 (males) and Figure 5–2 (females). Figure 5–3 and Figure 5–4 superimpose these growth curves over the CDC growth curves for the general population. It can be seen that the mean stature and weight for children with VCFS tend to run below that of the general population in infancy and early childhood. There are plateaus over months during which there is relatively little growth, followed by spurts of growth that bring the VCFS sample closer to the curve of the general population. The mean values for the VCFS sample approaches the mean for the general population in adolescence, and in adulthood the means are very close. It can be seen that weight tends to lag behind height when compared to CDC norms for all ages in childhood until early adolescence and the onset of puberty, when weight becomes proportionate to height for both boys and girls in relation to the CDC norms. However, as mentioned earlier, the CDC norms for the general population do not apply to children with VCFS, so the distribution of weight to height is different than for the general population.

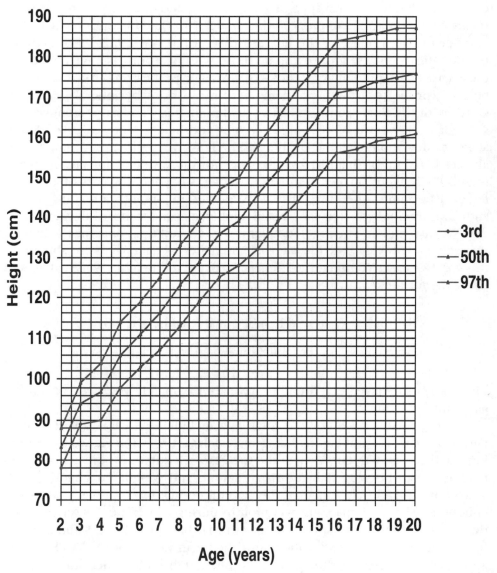

**2 to 20 years: boys, Height for age**

Legend: 3rd, 50th, 97th

**FIGURE 5–1.** Growth curves from birth to 20 years for males with VCFS including (a) height for age from 2 to 20 years; (b) length for age from birth to 36 months; (c) weight for age from 2 to 20 years; and (d) weight for age from birth to 36 months. *continues*

## Birth to 36 months: boys, length for age

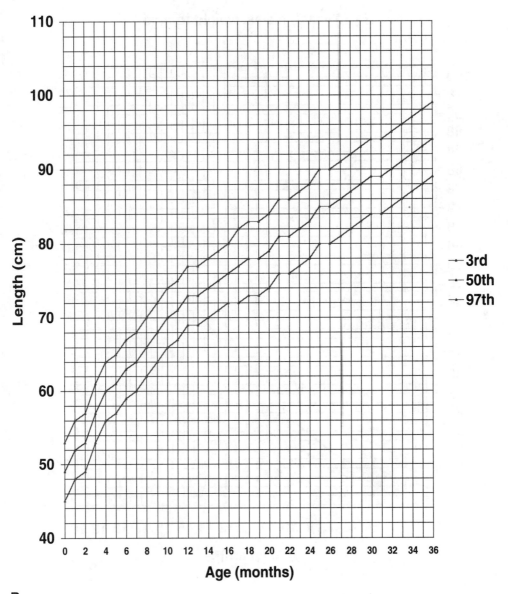

**B**

**FIGURE 5–1.** *continued*

# 2 - 20 years: males, weight for age

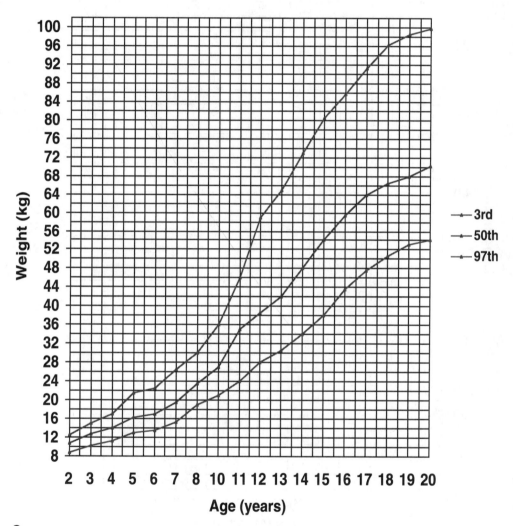

C

**FIGURE 5–1.** *continued*

## Birth to 36 months: boys, weight for age

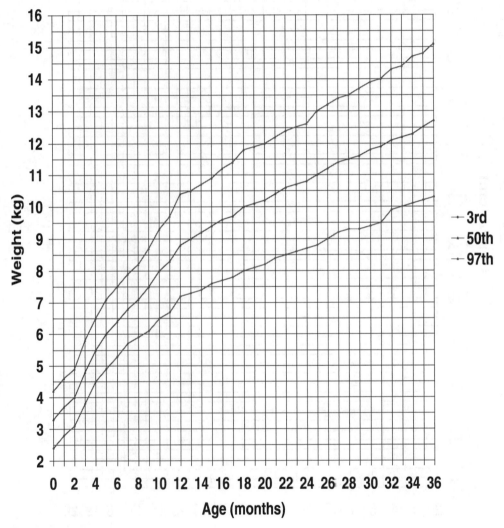

**D**

**FIGURE 5–1.** *continued*

# 2 - 20 years: girls, height for age

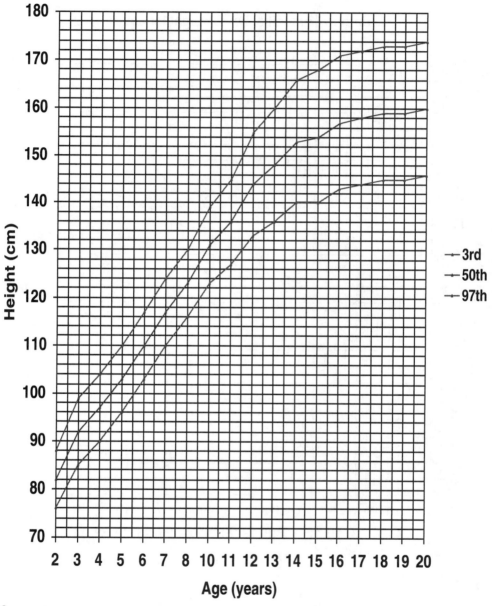

A

**FIGURE 5–2.** Growth curve from birth to 20 years for females with VCFS including (a) height for age from 2 to 20 years; (b) length for age from birth to 36 months; (c) weight for age from 2 to 20 years; and (d) weight for age from birth to 36 months. *continues*

# Birth to 36 months: girls, length for age

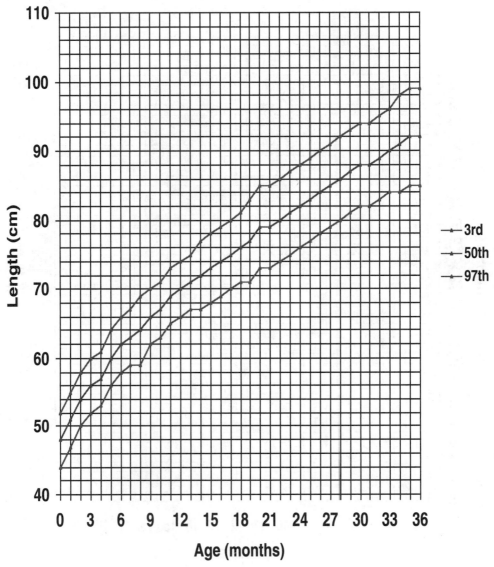

**B**

**FIGURE 5–2.** *continued*

## 2 - 20 years: females, weight for age

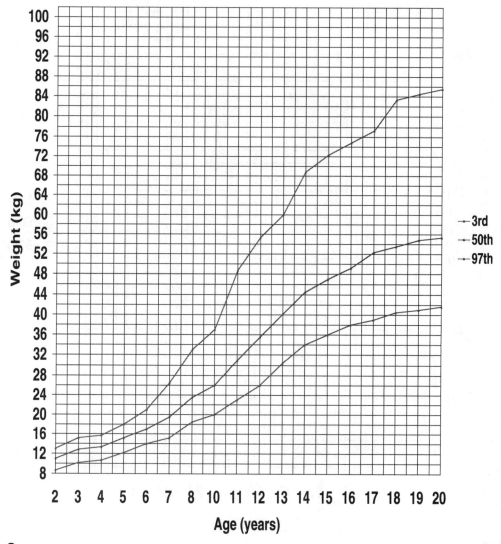

C

**FIGURE 5–2.** *continued*

# Birth to 36 months: girls, weight for age

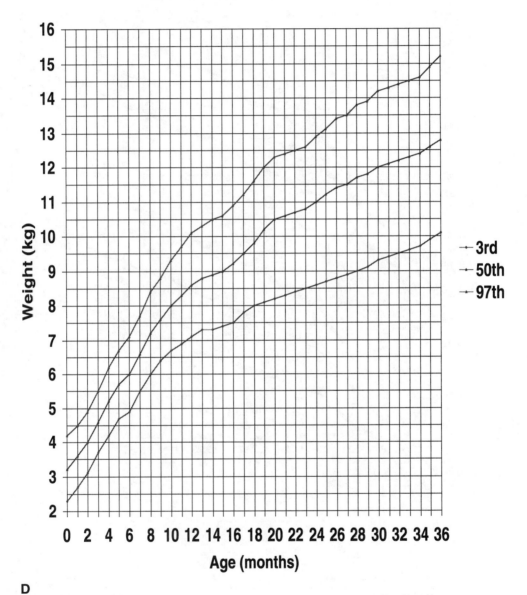

**D**

**FIGURE 5–2.** *continued*

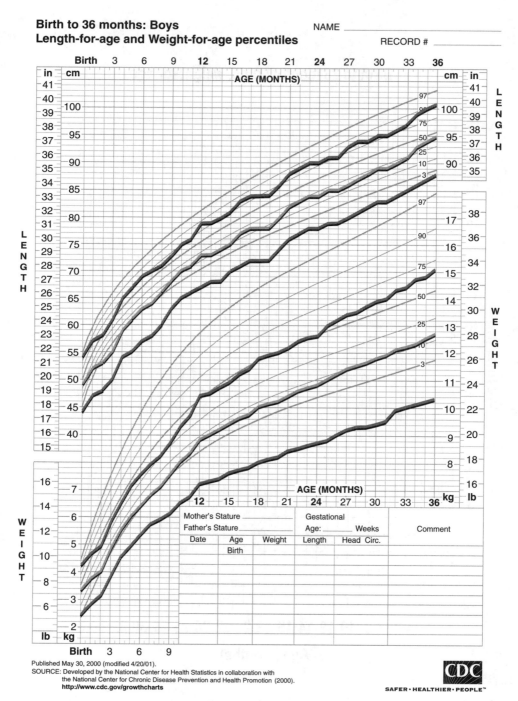

**Birth to 36 months: Boys**
**Length-for-age and Weight-for-age percentiles**

NAME _____

RECORD # _____

Published May 30, 2000 (modified 4/20/01).
SOURCE: Developed by the National Center for Health Statistics in collaboration with
the National Center for Chronic Disease Prevention and Health Promotion (2000).
http://www.cdc.gov/growthcharts

**FIGURE 5–3.** Growth curves from birth to 20 years for males with VCFS superimposed over the same curves for the general population as published by the CDC. The lines for VCFS include the 50th (*middle line*), 97th (*top line*), and 3rd centiles (*bottom line*). *Note.* From National Center for Health Statistics, 2000. Available from http://www.cdc.gov/growthcharts *continues*

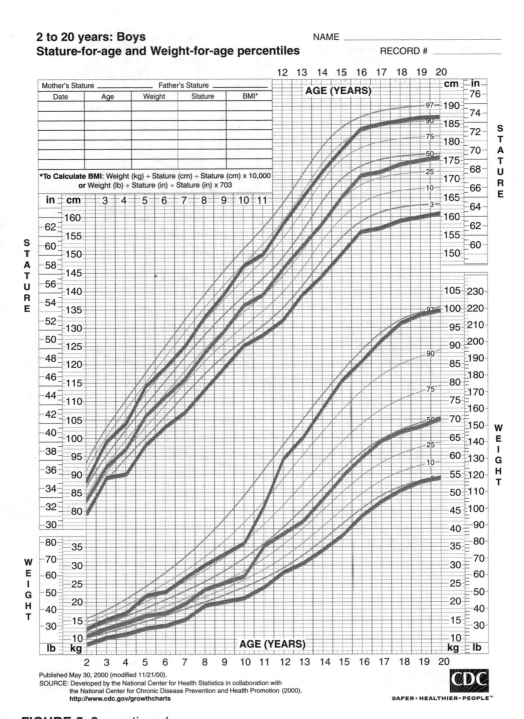

**2 to 20 years: Boys**
**Stature-for-age and Weight-for-age percentiles**

NAME _____

RECORD # _____

*To Calculate BMI: Weight (kg) ÷ Stature (cm) ÷ Stature (cm) x 10,000
or Weight (lb) ÷ Stature (in) ÷ Stature (in) x 703

Published May 30, 2000 (modified 11/21/00).
SOURCE: Developed by the National Center for Health Statistics in collaboration with
the National Center for Chronic Disease Prevention and Health Promotion (2000).
http://www.cdc.gov/growthcharts

**CDC**
SAFER·HEALTHIER·PEOPLE™

**FIGURE 5–3.** *continued*

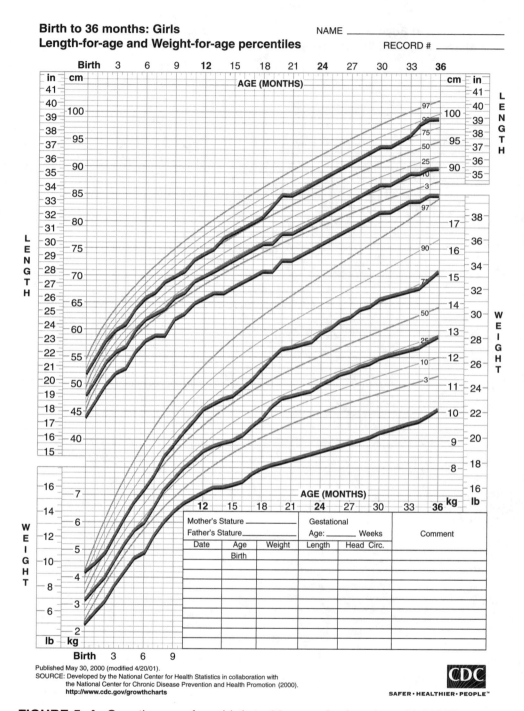

**Birth to 36 months: Girls**
**Length-for-age and Weight-for-age percentiles**

NAME _____

RECORD # _____

Published May 30, 2000 (modified 4/20/01).
SOURCE: Developed by the National Center for Health Statistics in collaboration with
the National Center for Chronic Disease Prevention and Health Promotion (2000).
http://www.cdc.gov/growthcharts

**FIGURE 5–4.** Growth curve from birth to 20 years for females with VCFS superimposed over the same curves for the general population as published by the CDC. *Note.* From National Center for Health Statistics, 2000. Available from http://www.cdc.gov/growthcharts *continues*

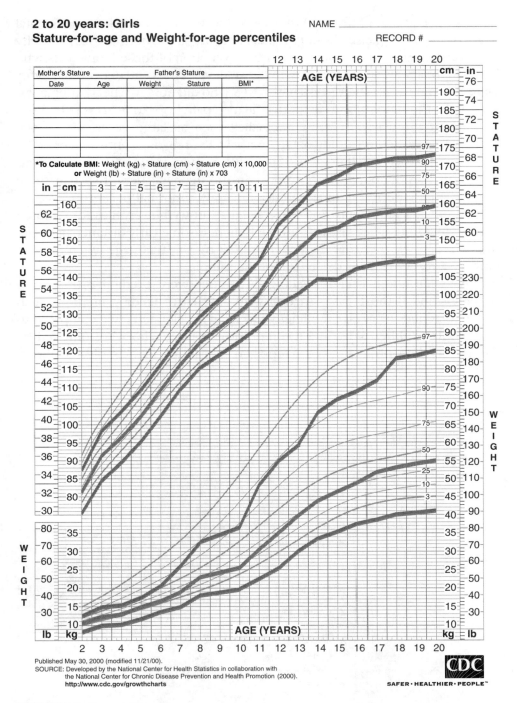

**2 to 20 years: Girls**
**Stature-for-age and Weight-for-age percentiles**

NAME _____

RECORD # _____

Published May 30, 2000 (modified 11/21/00).
SOURCE: Developed by the National Center for Health Statistics in collaboration with
the National Center for Chronic Disease Prevention and Health Promotion (2000).
http://www.cdc.gov/growthcharts

SAFER · HEALTHIER · PEOPLE™

**FIGURE 5–4.** *continued*

The separation of the growth data for those with and without congenital heart disease compared these two subpopulations for both growth velocity and eventual growth outcomes. With the exception of those individuals who had pulmonary atresia or stenosis, the growth velocities and expected heights were the same as for their peers with VCFS who did not have heart anomalies, except for the time prior to definitive heart repair. Prior to heart repair, those cases with more severe heart anomalies such as large ventricular septal defects lagged behind other babies with VCFS, but only until surgery. The majority of cases of tetralogy of Fallot, interrupted aortic arch, and truncus arteriosus had definitive heart surgery in the neonatal period so that there was not a long period of time with significantly abnormal perfusion.

Figure 5–5 and Figure 5–6 show height and weight profiles for children with and without heart disease. Although there is some early distance between the two samples, these are no longer present by 3 years of age when the pulmonary atresia cases are deleted from the sample.

We then asked if early feeding difficulties were predictive of growth problems and if those cases treated with alternative feeding methods such as gastrostomies or gavage feedings grew at an accelerated pace compared to other VCFS children who had feeding problems but who were only fed by mouth. Feeding problems were reported in 74% of the sample. Of those,

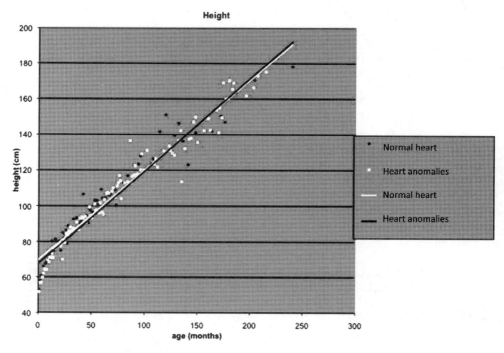

**FIGURE 5–5.** Height and weight profiles for males with VCFS with and without heart disease. Note that the trends for both coincide.

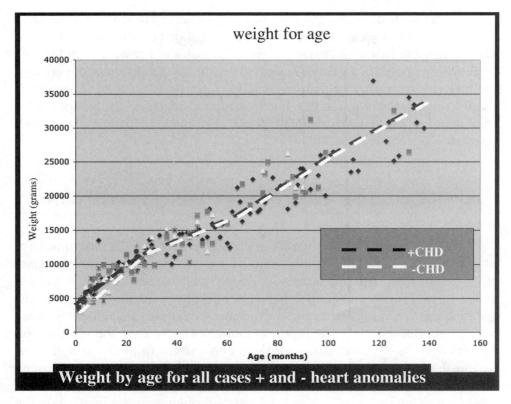

**FIGURE 5–6.** Height and weight profiles for females with VCFS with and without heart disease. Note that the trends for both coincide.

approximately one quarter were fed by gavage (nasogastric tubes) or gastrostomy (and its variations, including J-tubes). Almost all of these procedures were implemented for at least a year, and those with gastrostomies had them for a mean period of 3 years, ranging from 1 to 7 years. When the growth velocities of the children with alternative feeding procedures were compared to the rest of the sample, there was no difference in growth velocity or eventual outcome. We also looked at the cases with reported failure to thrive or feeding difficulties and compared them to the entire VCFS sample and also found no differences in growth velocity.

We then assessed the expected heights for the 127 adults. We found that 92% of the males in the sample were within 3 cm of their calculated expected heights. The distribution of those above expected height was essentially the same as those slightly below; three cases were within 3 cm below expected height, two were above. Of the remaining five males in the sample, one was 15 cm taller than expected, and four were between 3 cm and 7 cm shorter than expected. Of these shorter cases, three had no heart disease, and three had histories of long-term G-tube placement.

The females in the sample did not reach expected height with the same frequency as the males and tended to be a bit shorter than their peers, but less than one standard deviation. Of the 67 females in the adult sample, 74% were within 3 cm of calculated expected height, and of those who were not, the majority were shorter than expected height. None were of severe short stature (below the 3rd centile), but a sizeable portion of the sample, 10%, were at or below the 10th centile for general population norms and were well below their predicted heights.

## SIGNIFICANCE OF THESE DATA AND THE GROWTH CURVE

We have seen many children with VCFS who have had life-altering operative procedures in infancy and childhood that have had a major impact on quality of life. Major traumatic procedures seen repeatedly in children with VCFS are gastrostomies and jejunostomies, Nissen fundal plications, and long-term gavage feedings by nasogastric tubes. Application of these procedures is based on a number of incorrect assumptions about VCFS. The first and most important relates to the growth curve for VCFS constructed from our sample. Low weight does not equate with failure to thrive. Weight in VCFS falls substantially below the normative data for the general population reflected by the CDC growth charts for infants and children, although it approximates it in the general population by teen years. Height is also less for boys and girls with VCFS until adolescence, although not as low as weight when compared to general population norms. Of course, it is always important to measure linear growth in children every time they are weighed, but weight–to-height ratios for VCFS are not comparable to population normal. Children with VCFS have primary hypotonia and have less muscle mass than children who do not have the deletion. Muscle is a very heavy tissue both because of its cellular density and because of its rich blood supply. It is much heavier than fat and connective tissue per cubic centimeter. When muscle mass is reduced, body weight is very low. We have seen many children labeled as having failure to thrive or poor weight gain yet who have fat on their abdomens, thighs, arms, and necks (Figure 5–7). Children do not deposit fat under their skin unless they are getting enough calories to support linear growth. Excess calories are stored as fat. Therefore, regardless of the numerical values on a scale and a stadiometer, clinicians must use their eyes and common sense to determine if a child is not getting enough calories to support growth.

Often, when a child refuses more food during a feeding, it is because his stomach is full and he has consumed all of the calories he wants and needs. Putting more food into him will only induce spitting up, emesis, and discomfort. Overfeeding is particularly problematic in VCFS because the chronic constipation encountered in many children with VCFS prevents the stomach from emptying at a normal pace. The discomfort will lead to an unhappy feed-

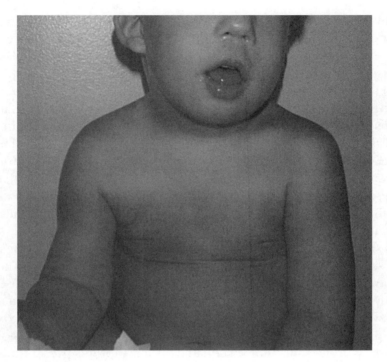

**FIGURE 5–7.** Photos of a 6-month-old child with VCFS labeled as having failure to thrive because of low weight and low weight to height proportion. Note that he has significant subcutaneous fat, including fat on his hands, on his arms, and around his belly.

ing situation and stress on both the parents and the child. If these findings result in the recommendation for a fundal plication or G-tube, the child is then made medically dependent, and the entire dynamic of the family is changed by removing pleasant mealtimes from the daily routine. Moreover, babies who are fed by tube never learn that the way to satiate hunger is to eat something. They are fed by a tube on schedule and never have the pleasurable experience of tasting food and pairing the act of eating with eliminating hunger pangs. The longer they stay on tube feedings, the more difficult it is to teach them to eat and to allow them the pleasure of eating. Also, clinicians must be aware that the family interaction that happens during mealtimes is one that is filled with conversation, language stimulation, social interaction, and a great deal of happiness for most families. An enormous amount of learning happens during family meals, including the art of conversation. Could the absence of these times in a child's life further impair language development?

Another misconception is that frequent emesis in infancy and childhood is actually reflux and that nasal reflux (which is simply emesis coming through the nose) puts a child at risk for aspiration and pneumonia. Carried one step further, pneumonia in VCFS is presumed to be aspiration pneumonia, especially when the child is having feeding difficulties and persistent emesis. Nasal emesis is not correlated in any way to aspiration. Furthermore, in most instances, pneumonia in children with VCFS is related to immune issues and not to aspiration. Unfortunately, the language used to describe spitting up (emesis) as "reflux" leads the clinician to believe that the problem is one of GER or GERD, which leads to specific treatments. When medications fail, fundal plications are often recommended. If the child also has low weight in relation to the CDC norms and it is not possible to increase weight with oral feedings, and if the child feeds to a point and then refuses more food, gastrostomies are often recommended. Hyperalimentation is then attempted through a G-tube or J-tube, and with the Nissen fundal plication in place, the child is unable to vomit when the stomach is overfilled. When this occurs, the child experiences persistent episodes of retching, often violent retching. The stomach empties slowly, especially with most children with VCFS being constipated, causing significant abdominal discomfort; the child does not want to eat by mouth because he does not feel hunger and in fact feels abdominal discomfort.

Although these issues were discussed within the context of specific anomalies in Chapter 2, they deserve repetition in the context of growth and the data presented here. Clinicians must be aware that the problems observed in children with VCFS cannot be equated with symptoms present in the general population. When problems go unexplained in VCFS, clinicians may be tempted to seek exotic explanations and exotic treatments that are major disruptions in the life of the patient and the family. If clinical experience showed us that these explanations were accurate and the treatments were effective, then they could be supported. However, just the opposite is true. The first step is the careful assessment of the patient's phenotype, followed by the inferential and deductive analysis of the symptoms in relation to these anomalies. In other words, before recommending a fundal plication for persistent emesis, ask why it is occurring in relation to the phenotypic findings. Try to be certain that the treatment is not worse than the disease, and try to be certain that the assessment of risk is real.

## POSSIBLE FLAWS IN THE DATA

Assembling the growth curve presented in this chapter was a complicated process involving years of data collection. That being said, there are some possible flaws in the curves that are related to the data used and how they were obtained. The most obvious problem is the lack of standardization in obtaining heights and weights. There is enormous variation in how anthropometric data are obtained, the accuracy of equipment, and the amount of clothing the child has on when weighed. Obviously, there are many variables that would affect the data collection process. We do not have any reason to suspect that the number of overestimates of weight outnumber the underestimates, but there certainly might be an effect on each individual data point and the standard deviation calculation for that age range.

Although these data represent a large data set for a rare disorder, the sample is still relatively small for constructing a growth curve. For many of the months of age we had hundreds of data points. For birth weight, we had over 1000 data points and the early years of life provided large numbers per month of age. Late adolescent and adult measures were lower in number, with some months having only a dozen or so data points, which makes the calculations less robust and standard deviations larger. When dealing with retrospective data of this type, we have to take what is available. We may also be dealing with a biased sample. It is possible that the mildest cases of VCFS, in other words, the most normal people, are never diagnosed, or if they are diagnosed but are not symptomatic for any major problems, they may have no reason to visit our center and therefore would be excluded from the study. Another issue that could affect linear growth is scoliosis. Scoliosis occurs in approximately 30% of individuals with VCFS, although it is often mild. Scoliosis will reduce linear growth measurements. Although our sample of individuals with scoliosis was essentially equally divided between males and females, we cannot calculate relative severity and effect on height. However, if anything, the sample may be skewed to a lower growth velocity than in the general population because of some degree of loss of height in approximately 30% of the sample.

## IMPLICATIONS

It is now clear that the reason earlier reports cited short stature as a feature of VCFS was because individual cases were compared in a cross-sectional manner to normative data for the general population. Growth velocity differs for VCFS in terms of the timing and periodic velocity, but not in terms of total growth. People with VCFS are not abnormally small when they reach adult life; they simply reach their adult height at a different pace than other people. This points out the need to follow populations of rare conditions over time in order to understand eventual outcomes and prognoses.

Except in early infancy until definitive heart surgery, the presence of CHD was not a factor in long-term growth, with the exception of severe cases of pulmonary atresia or stenosis. The poor peripheral perfusion that occurs with pulmonary atresia limits growth because there is not sufficient drive to stimulate the formation of new peripheral blood vessels. Definitive repair of heart anomalies did not impair the long-term outcome in relation to expected height. Males reached expected heights, females tended to fall slightly short by comparison, but severe short stature was not seen in either males or females.

In childhood, weight was low compared to height (typically between the 10th to 25th centile) for individuals with VCFS. However, this discrepancy was common and independent of eating habits or diagnosis of failure to thrive. Many children had weight-to-height proportions at or below the 10th centile yet still had normal or even excessive amounts of body fat. Evidence indicates that muscle mass is reduced in VCFS (Zim et al., 2003) and that muscle fibers are smaller than normal. It seems likely that the weight-to-height and body mass indices calculated for children in the general population are not relevant to children with VCFS. After puberty, weight increased relative to height, but examination of these children showed that many appear overweight with disproportionate amounts of body fat. The reason for this is not clear. It may be related to hypotonia and lower activity levels or perhaps to hypothyroidism, a common finding in adolescence. It may also be that changes in the endocrine system may prompt weight gain more than in the general population.

Early feeding difficulties were not predictive of short stature or low weight as an adolescent or adult. More important, the use of alternative feeding in infancy did not increase linear growth velocity. Those individuals who had major surgical procedures related to feeding such as fundal plication and gastrostomy did not have an advantage in long-term or short-term growth over those who struggled with feeding but did not have surgery.

The conclusion drawn from these data is simple. The one factor that had an effect on how children with VCFS grow is the deletion. Feeding difficulties, heart anomalies (with the exception of pulmonary atresia), treatments, diet, history of illness, and all other factors did not have an effect on long-term outcome. VCFS is not a syndrome of short stature. This should not come as a surprise. Children with many, if not most, multiple anomaly syndromes have abnormal growth patterns compared to the general population. The overwhelming majority of people with chromosomal rearrangements involving multiple genes have abnormal growth patterns, and the large majority of them have deficient growth velocity. Comparing these people to growth charts based on the general population in order to recommend treatment is not appropriate. Once the diagnosis of VCFS is made, all treatment decisions and all parameters of growth and development need to be placed within the context of the diagnosis. Treatments need to be implemented based on outcomes, especially treatments that will have a major impact on quality of life.

## FEEDING THERAPY

Unfortunately, when clinicians feel they have no other option, or they are unable to understand the issues related to how VCFS affects feeding, they recommend surgical alternatives to feeding and placement of tubes in the stomach or jejunum for feeding and to allow the baby to gain weight. On occasion, this approach may be an expedient approach to having children discharged from hospitals so that they are not inpatients for a protracted period of time while they are taught to eat. Expedient solutions are not typically ideal solutions, and the reality is that given the proper knowledge base, some time and patience, and appropriate diagnostic and treatment protocols, feeding should be accomplished successfully in nearly all patients with VCFS.

If the major effect on growth is the deletion and the outcomes from treatment do not make any difference in long-term prognosis, then what should be done? The first answer is, "Don't panic." The presentations that cause major concern in babies with VCFS are emesis (often mislabeled as reflux, as discussed earlier in this chapter and in Chapter 2) and prolonged feeding time with little success. These are two separate issues in VCFS.

### Emesis and Spitting Up Through the Nose

The first challenge is to find out why the emesis or tiring is occurring. In terms of emesis, the first step is to stop calling it reflux, or if it is coming out of the nose, nasal reflux. The reason emesis may occur through the nose is VPI and because the large volume of the nasopharynx is the path of least resistance. The cause for the emesis and spitting up through the nose include:

1. Vascular ring or other vascular compression of the esophagus

2. Chronic constipation, slow gastric emptying, and attempts to hyperaliment

3. Chronic stimulation of a laryngeal adductor reflex by contact of another structure with the aryepiglottic fold

4. Too much air becoming entrapped in the esophagus or stomach

Although each of these factors may cause emesis and spitting up individually, they may also occur additively. They are not mutually exclusive.

1. Tiring during feeding is related to a number of factors, as well:
   Congenital heart disease

2. Hypotonia

3. Hypocalcemia

4. Chronic illness from an immune disorder

5. Airway compromise from Robin sequence, retrognathia, or hypotonia

All of these factors may cause or contribute to lethargy, lack of vigor, and reduced strength. It is therefore important to reduce the amount of work needed to extract milk into the mouth.

There are some general feeding techniques that are useful to use uniformly in babies with VCFS. They involve time, position, the type of bottle and nipple, and burping (Sidoti & Shprintzen, 1995). In most cases, breastfeeding is not possible with babies with VCFS because it is difficult for them to extract milk from the breast in terms of suction and strength. Although some babies with VCFS can nurse successfully, most cannot. We prefer bottle-feeding if there is any question about failure to nurse well. This way we can reduce effort on the part of the baby and we can also track how much the baby is taking.

### Feeding Time (Duration)

When a baby is feeding poorly, each feeding may last for 45 minutes or an hour. This is far too long, especially for a baby with congenital heart disease. The baby will tire easily and may be expending more calories in the feeding process than are being taken in from the bottle. We instruct parents to try to limit the feeding to 20 minutes, 30 at the most, but no more than 30 minutes. We recommend a 3-hour schedule for neonates that can then be lengthened to 4 hours in several weeks if successful and there is more oral intake per feeding. Once there is no difficulty with the feeding process, demand feedings can be instituted. If feedings take a long time, the baby will be awake and expending energy for a long time. Babies actually gain weight when they are asleep and their metabolism slows, allowing their calories to be put to good use for growth rather than burned in the amount of energy it takes to feed. When on a schedule, we would like to lengthen the time between feedings so the baby is hungry at the next feeding. In this way, the infant will pair the stimulus of feeding to the comfortable feeling of satiation, thus reinforcing the feeding process. As part of the time issue, we teach the parents to look at the bottle during the feeding to make sure they are seeing air bubbles enter the bottle from the nipple (Figure 5–8). The presence of air bubbles indicates that milk is leaving the bottle and being replaced by air (in response to the

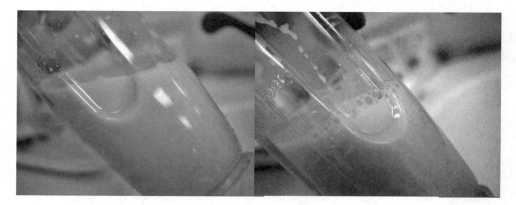

**FIGURE 5–8.** A bottle filled with formula at the beginning of feeding (*left*) and then during feeding (*right*). Note the air bubbles entering the bottle indicating that milk has exited the bottle and is being replaced by air. This is a positive sign that the baby is feeding well.

negative pressure in the bottle) and is a good sign that the baby is feeding well. If air bubbles are not entering the bottle, then the feeding is not being successful and feeding technique needs to be altered.

## Feeding Position

Babies with VCFS should be held in as upright a position as possible during feeding. This will allow gravity to assist in the passage of food from the pharynx to the esophagus, and gravity will prevent pooling in the pyriforms and cricopharyngeus. Should emesis or spitting up occur, there is less risk that the vomitus will pool in the pharynx, thus decreasing the risk of aspiration.

If the baby has a cleft that extends into the hard palate, the tip of the nipple should be held to one side of the palate or the other so that the contents of the bottle do not go directly into the cleft and out of the nose. The baby will not care of the tip is lateral to the midline.

## Type of Bottle and Nipple

There are many types of feeding implements available. Our preference is a clear bottle with a soft, squeezable side and a soft nipple with a large hole. Two widely available bottle/nipple sets are the Abbott Nutrition Similac Premature Nipple (often referred to as the Ross red premie nipple). This is attached to the Ross soft squeeze bottle (Figure 5–9). This nipple has a small cross-cut at the tip, so the flow is a bit faster than a normal rubber nipple, but it may not be as fast as needed for a baby with significant hypotonia or with a palatal anomaly. Therefore, we typically enlarge the cross-cut to allow a larger volume to be extracted from the nipple with each suck. The baby might initially be surprised by the increase in flow and might cough or choke. Some people become alarmed when this happens but should not be. This is actually a normal response and a good sign that the baby can protect the airway. Give the baby a moment to recover and then reinsert the bottle. After several feedings, the baby will learn to adjust the flow by varying the amount of pressure he puts on the nipple with the tongue. If the baby becomes tired during the feeding before finishing, or if there is still not a sufficiently rapid flow of fluid, the bottle can be gently squeezed to push out additional fluid. Babies drink and swallow during sleep or drowsiness without any difficulty.

Another bottle and nipple similar to the Ross system is the Enfamil Cleft Lip/Palate Nurser (Figure 5–10). The Enfamil setup works exactly the same way as the Ross units and works just as well. In cases where a baby is very weak or hypotonic, we have found the Soft-Sipp system works well because it does require sucking; it works more like a syringe by directly injecting milk into the baby's mouth (Figure 5–11). If special bottles and nipples are not available, most nipples can be modified by cutting larger holes and softened by boiling them several times. Plastic bottles that can be squeezed can also be found in most markets and pharmacies.

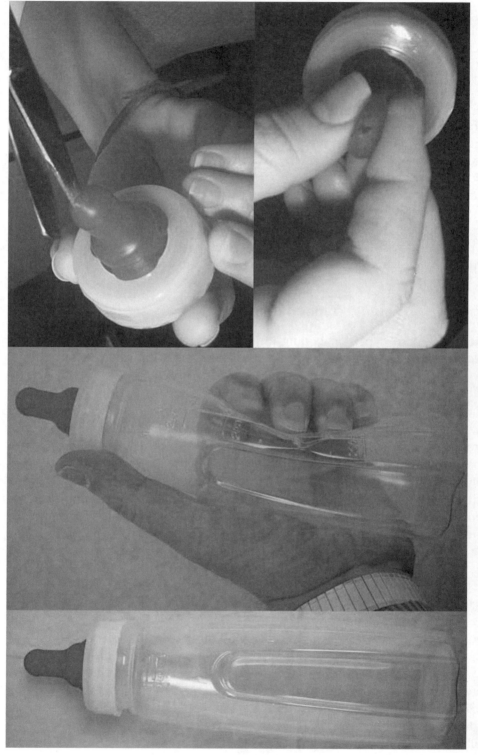

**FIGURE 5–9.** Similac premie nipple attached to Ross soft squeeze bottle and showing enlargement of the cross cut in the nipple.

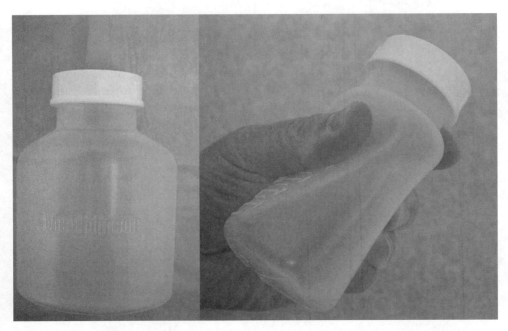

**FIGURE 5–10.** Enfamil Cleft Lip/Cleft Palate feeder with a soft, squeezable bottle.

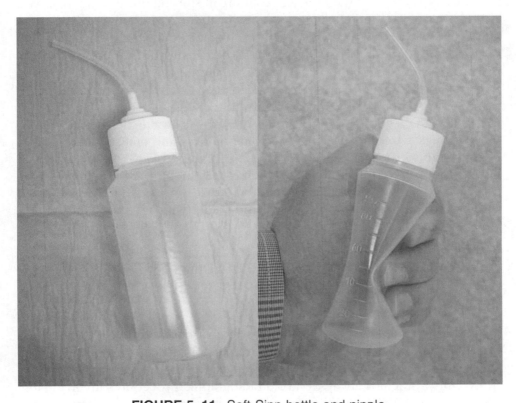

**FIGURE 5–11.** Soft-Sipp bottle and nipple.

The use of these implements, although they are not the only ones that could be used, has the intent of reducing effort while maximizing the delivery time of the food. If the mother is capable of expressing her own milk, this is the preferred food. In cases where this is not possible, formula can be fed in the same manner. Once the baby grows and is stronger, there is no longer the need to use special implements or techniques. In rare cases, it may be necessary to use nasogastric gavage feedings temporarily. This might be necessary before and after heart surgery in babies with severe anomalies and dramatically reduced strength and perfusion, but once heart surgery has corrected some or all of the perfusion issues, every attempt should be made to establish oral feedings and normalize life.

## Burping

Babies who have a difficult time creating suction for easy feeding have to suck more often to get a sufficient bolus to swallow. During the sucking efforts, they are breathing through their noses. The more breathing that happens during feeding, the more air they are likely to swallow with their food. Air entrapped in the esophagus or stomach will eventually come out, often as burps that might carry some food with the air, resulting in spitting up. Too much air will also likely create discomfort and potentially abdominal cramping. The problem will be worse in babies who are constipated because the air could become entrapped in the digestive tract. To prevent the amount of air from being too large, babies with VCFS should be burped every few minutes, rather than the normal several times during a feeding. If the baby does not burp after a minute or so, then the baby can return to feeding.

When the feeding is completed, if the baby is awake, he should be kept upright for a while in case there is going to be some emesis. This is often a good time to socially engage the child, and a good way is to have him as upright as possible in an infant seat facing the parent. If emesis occurs, simply clean it up and do not feed the child more. It is possible that the stomach cannot hold any more food because of slow emptying and overfilling.

## IDENTIFYING AND UNDERSTANDING THE FACTORS LEADING TO PROBLEMS

It should be possible to rule out or discover a vascular ring by echocardiography. Other diagnostic tests could include esophagoscopy, MR scan of the chest including MR angiography, CT scan of the chest, or barium swallow study. Our protocol is always to avoid radiographic procedures involving ionizing radiation if there are alternatives. The echocardiogram would be the first choice, followed by either the MR scan or esophagoscopy. The barium swallow study irradiates the neck and thyroid, often for prolonged periods, and the quality of the information with respect to vascular compression is difficult to interpret. In fact, if it looked like there was an esophageal stricture that might be vascular in nature, the next step would be to order an ultrasound or MR scan. CT scanning should certainly be avoided because of the high radiation levels involved, even with modern scanners. If a vascular ring is discovered, then it is likely that this will require surgical correction, especially if it is causing respiratory compromise. If there is no vascular ring, there may be compression of the esophagus by an aberrant vessel, such as a subclavian artery or an abnormal course of the aorta. If the esophagus is being compressed, then a bolus of food will get hung up in the esophagus just above the stricture. The response of the esophagus will be to get rid of it by a reverse peristalsis if it cannot be cleared rapidly enough to be swallowed. Therefore, what is coming up in this type of emesis is not food that has been completely swallowed, but food that has been almost swallowed. Because this problem is typically occurring at the stage where babies are drinking only milk (mother's milk or formula), it is not really possible to thin the food too much to ease it through the point of compression. What is the solution? Again, the first step is not to panic. Although there might be a slight risk of aspiration following emesis, it should not be a major risk if the baby is neurologically intact with a normal laryngeal adductor reflex, normal cough, and no evidence of an adductor paralysis of the larynx. Although laryngeal paralysis and paresis can occur in VCFS, true paralysis is rare, and the failure to adduct the vocal cords is also rare. FEES can be used to rule out aspiration. The solution to a narrowing of the esophagus by compression of a single artery is usually time. With growth and expansion of the chest, the problem will gradually improve and resolve. The challenge therefore becomes knowing that the baby has fed enough. This can be measured by checking for a normal amount of urination and eyeballing the baby to make sure that he is maintaining body fat. Parents should try to remain calm during periods of emesis because adding anxiety to the feeding situation will be transmitted to the baby in short order. The feeding process will become unpleasant and frustrating for all concerned. If the baby is thriving, behaving reasonably well, enjoys the feeding process, and is maintaining body fat, then simply wipe up the vomitus and move on.

Chronic constipation is very common in VCFS and typically contributes substantially to feeding difficulties. The basic principle is that if food is not clearing out of one end, you cannot put it in the other end. Chronic constipation will make the baby feel full and uncomfortable so that there is no hunger or appetite. There may also be abdominal cramping. If the parent tries to force the baby to eat under these circumstances, the feeding situation will take on very unpleasant emotional content and the baby will want to avoid mealtimes. Although it is not uncommon for some babies to go for several days without a bowel movement, there is a risk in VCFS that the stool will become so hard that it will be difficult to expel and cause even more pain. We therefore recommend being fairly aggressive in treating constipation in babies with VCFS. We would like to see at least one bowel movement per day (neonates and infants typically have three or more), and if the baby has not moved his or her bowels in two days, we recommend inducing a bowel movement. First attempts at inducing a bowel movement may be external stimulation of the rectum with a gentle stream of warm water or a warm washcloth, but if there is no response, a suppository and then eventually laxatives may become necessary based on advice from the baby's physician.

Constant stimulation of the aryepiglottic folds is also common in VCFS and can cause coughing, choking, and gagging. As discussed in Chapter 2, the pharynx is abnormal in a number of ways in VCFS. There may be significant asymmetry so that the entire posterior pharyngeal wall juts out on one side (Figure 5–12). One immediate effect is to compromise the pyriform on that side, partially blocking the path of a bolus that could penetrate the laryngeal vestibule and cause choking or coughing. The other is to make direct contact with the aryepiglottic fold, prompting a laryngeal adductor reflex resulting in gagging, choking, or breath-holding.

Another phenomenon observed in infants and children with VCFS is that an ectopic and medialized internal carotid artery can be so prominent as to persistently stimulate the aryepiglottic fold, with the same effect of coughing,

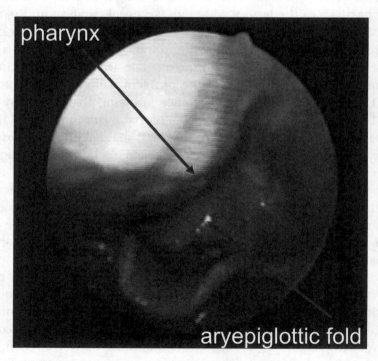

**FIGURE 5–12.** Prominence of one side of the pharynx in an asymmetric hypopharynx, causing direct contact with the aryepiglottic fold and chronic coughing and gagging in a child with VCFS.

gagging, and choking (see Video 2–16, the fourth case shown). The stimulation of the aryepiglottic folds by the pharyngeal wall or the internal carotid is something that will resolve with age, albeit gradually. It is critical that these problems not be assumed or surmised. Both are easily diagnosed by fiberoptic endoscopy with the patient awake and held upright in the same position used for feeding.

As infants with VCFS get older and approach their first birthday, another source of persistent stimulation of the aryepiglottic folds and the epiglottis is hypertrophic tonsils (see Video 2–9). As discussed in Chapter 2, hypertrophic tonsils that grow posteriorly and inferiorly into the hypopharyngeal airway are common in VCFS and can only be diagnosed by fiberoptic endoscopy. Per-oral examination will not reveal this problem.

Airway issues are often responsible for feeding difficulties in VCFS, as is also true for many other craniofacial disorders. In some cases, there is obvious evidence of upper airway obstruction with observed apneas, and if this is the case, oral feeding will be essentially impossible to accomplish. With an already compromised airway, putting a bottle or food into a baby's mouth will only serve to compromise the airway more. Babies will always preserve respiration as a first priority. Babies with upper airway obstruction will struggle during feeding and will seem to avoid the nipple. They will cry, get agitated, impound air in the esophagus because of their struggle to breathe, and will have substernal, suprasternal, and intercostal retractions (see Video 2–14). In babies with VCFS who have Robin sequence, this type of feeding problem is ubiquitous. It is essential to resolve the airway problem in order to solve the feeding problem. On occasion, airway problems will resolve over time. In such cases, gavage feedings for a period of weeks may be indicated to allow the baby to rest and grow. Because the mandible in VCFS is structurally normal, it is not typically necessary to surgically advance it by distraction, something that is commonly done for other infants with Robin sequence who do not have VCFS. Tracheotomies are rarely necessary.

## WHAT IF THE CHILD ALREADY HAS A TUBE?

Establishing normal feeding after the child has already had long-term alternative feeding techniques (gavage or surgical) is more difficult than establishing normal feeding practices in infancy. The child may have gone years without tasting food, or if he is taking small amounts by mouth, without being able to understand the pleasure of eating in relation to satiation and the social aspects of meals. In addition, if the child has had a fundal plication and the normally low weight associated with VCFS prompts the recommendation for hyperalimentation, there will be significant discomfort from overfilling of the digestive tract; the food cannot escape through the esophagus in the form of emesis or spitting up, and because the stomach empties slowly, the overfilling often prompts retching in an attempt to vomit, which is not possible because of the fundal plication.

Based on referrals to us of children who have been in feeding therapy, it seems that the most popular approach among current clinicians is the use of "oral-motor therapy" or "oral-motor stimulation." Clinicians will often use a variety of implements like soft brushes, glycerin swabs, and plastic devices to stimulate the mouth and oral musculature, as if this was going to induce eating behavior. We have also encountered clinicians who employ oral and facial massage, both external and internal, including rubbing of the lips, tongue, and even the palate. These procedures abound even in the absence of scientific outcome data that demonstrate effectiveness. In fact, based on histories from parents whose children have been exposed to these procedures, it is clear that the children find them annoying, as would anyone in the same circumstances. These procedures make no sense and should not be applied. Children who have not eaten for a long time need to be taught to eat. They must learn it. No amount of oral stimulation will make it happen, nor will such stimulation "set the stage" for the child to learn how to eat.

Eating is a volitional operant behavior. Swallowing, the actual transport of food through the esophagus into the stomach, is not volitional at all. Children do not have to be taught to swallow. Even if being fed by gastrostomy, they have been swallowing their saliva. Once food reaches the cricopharyngeus, there is a reflexive, brainstem mediated opening of the upper esophageal sphincter and the swallow occurs. Everything that happens prior to that point is not reflexive, but rather volitional behavior under control of the brain's cortex. Many learning theory advocates believe that the best learning is the learning that happens by trial and error. If the child puts things into his mouth, or if there is finger or thumb sucking behavior, a trial and error learning experience can be constructed by putting food, especially soft and pureed food, on a tray in front of the child in a high chair if the child is able to sit, or in an infant seat if the child needs support. Eventually the child will either play with the food with his hands or accidentally stick a hand into the food. The food should be highly flavored. If the child has already demonstrated an affinity for a particular flavor, use it. If not, put either sweet, salty, or savory food on the tray, like a vanilla or chocolate pudding, spaghetti sauce, or some melted ice cream. At this point, do not be concerned with nutritional value. The intent is simply to get the child interested in putting food in the mouth and tasting it. As soon as the child does so, the parent or caregiver should reinforce it immediately by praising the child or hugging the child or doing something that the child finds pleasurable, so the child will be more likely to repeat the behavior. Once the child has shown interest in repeatedly putting some food in his mouth, then the food stimuli can be varied. It will also be possible to engage the child in a game by letting the child see the food being put on the table with a spoon and seeing if the child will be interested in licking the spoon. This can be encouraged by having the parent lick the spoon first while showing great delight. As the child becomes willing to allow food to go into the mouth, new food stimuli can be introduced, again with the focus being on highly flavored foods, not necessarily nutritional content. As more food is taken orally, then more flavors and foods can be tried.

Drinking fluids can be done the same way. Highly flavored liquids can be chosen, like grape juice, chocolate milk, or a flavored milkshake. Small straws can be placed on the tray in front of the child with some of the liquid in the straws. Pieces of clean sponge too large to swallow can be soaked in the liquid and left on the tray. If the child puts these in the mouth, then some of the liquid will go into the mouth as well. Small cups can also be used for the child who can lift and manipulate them. The goal is to let the child's own behavior lead to the liquid being consumed. Once the child engages in putting things in the mouth, the parent can copy the behavior, and then eventually the child will allow the parent to deliver the liquid.

Changes in flavors should be made in small steps. It is possible to flavor foods and drinks in innovative ways so that the basic likes of the child can be matched. Children with VCFS do not accept rapid change well, so very gradual introductions of new foods and liquids should be made.

This type of trial and error learning will allow the child to engage in the learning process in a pleasurable way. If the child has previously been reluctant to have utensils and objects placed in his mouth, then the last thing one wants to do is to feed the child involuntarily and put things in the child's mouth that are not welcome.

**Acknowledgments.** We would like to thank the members of the Velo-Cardio-Facial Syndrome Educational Foundation, Inc. who responded to our call for data and took the time to send us information that constituted a major percentage of the information in this chapter. We would also like to thank the patients at the VCFS International Center, Department of Otolaryngology, State University of New York Upstate Medical University, Syracuse, NY, for their meticulous collection of records that permitted us to extract the necessary information in this chapter.

# REFERENCES

Motzkin, B., Marion, R., Goldberg, R., Shprintzen, R. J., & Saenger, P. (1993). Variable phenotypes in velocardiofacial syndrome with chromosomal deletion. *Journal of Pediatrics, 123,* 406–410.

Shprintzen, R. J., Goldberg, R. B., Lewin, M. L., Sidoti, E. J., Berkman, M. D., Argamaso, R. V., et al. (1978). A new syndrome involving cleft palate, cardiac anomalies, typical facies, and learning disabilities: Velo-cardio-facial syndrome. *Cleft Palate Journal, 15,* 56–62.

Sidoti, E. J., & Shprintzen, R. J. (1995). Pediatric care and feeding of the newborn with a cleft. In R. J. Shprintzen & J. Bardach (Eds.), *Cleft palate speech management: A multidisciplinary approach* (pp. 63–74). St. Louis, MO: Mosby.

Young, D., Shprintzen, R. J., & Goldberg, R. (1980). Cardiac malformations in the velo-cardio-facial syndrome. *American Journal of Cardiology, 46,* 43–48.

Zim, S., Schelper, R., Kellman, R., Tatum, S., Ploutz-Snyder, R., & Shprintzen, R. J. (2003). Thickness and histologic and histochemical properties of the superior pharyngeal constrictor muscle in velocardiofacial syndrome. *Archives of Facial and Plastic Surgery, 5,* 503–507.

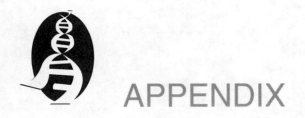 APPENDIX

# Clinical Synopsis of VCFS

1. Palate anomalies, including overt cleft palate, submucous cleft palate, occult submucous cleft palate, and asymmetric palate

2. Asymmetric pharynx

3. Platybasia

4. Retrognathia

5. Asymmetric crying facies (infancy)

6. Functional facial asymmetry

7. Structural facial asymmetry

8. Straight facial profile

9. Hypotonic facies

10. Vertical maxillary excess

11. Small primary teeth

12. Enamel hypoplasia (primary dentition)

13. Downturned oral commissures

14. Microstomia

15. Microcephaly

16. Small posterior cranial fossa

17. Cleft lip

18. Overfolded helix

19. Attached lobules

20. Protuberant, cup-shaped ears

21. Small ears

22. Mildly asymmetric ears

23. Frequent otitis media

24. Mild conductive hearing loss

25. Sensorineural hearing loss

26. Ear tags or pits

27. Narrow external ear canals

28. Prominent nasal bridge

29. Vertically long nose

30. Bulbous nasal tip

31. Mildly separated nasal domes (tip appears bifid)

32. Pinched alar base, narrow nostrils

33. Narrow nasal passages

34. Tortuous retinal vessels

35. Suborbital congestion ("allergic shiners")

36. Strabismus

37. Narrow palpebral fissures

38. Puffy upper eyelids

39. Small optic disk

40. Prominent corneal nerves

41. Cataract

42. Iris nodules

43. Iris coloboma (uncommon)

44. Retinal coloboma (uncommon)

45. Small eyes

46. Mild orbital hypertelorism

47. Mild vertical orbital dystopia

48. Posterior embryotoxon

49. Ventricular septal defect (VSD)

50. Atrial septal defect (ASD)

51. Pulmonic atresia or stenosis

52. Tetralogy of Fallot

53. Right-sided aorta

54. Vascular ring

55. Patent ductus arteriosus (PDA)

56. Interrupted aortic arch, type B

57. Coarctation of the aorta

58. Double aortic arch

59. Aortic valve anomalies

60. Aberrant subclavian arteries

61. Truncus arteriosus

62. Anomalous origin of carotid artery

63. Transposition of the great vessels

64. Tricuspid atresia

65. Medially displaced and/or ectopic internal carotid arteries

66. Tortuous or kinked internal carotids

67. Jugular vein anomalies

68. Absence of internal carotid artery (unilateral)

69. Absence of vertebral artery (unilateral)

70. Tortuous or kinked vertebral arteries

71. Low bifurcation of common carotid

72. Reynaud's phenomenon

73. Small veins

74. Circle of Willis anomalies

75. Reduced total brain volume

76. Variations in size of various brain segments, small cerebellar vermis, and cerebellar hypoplasia

77. Periventricular cysts

78. White matter hyperintensities

79. Generalized hypotonia

80. Cerebellar ataxia

81. Seizures

82. Strokes

83. Spina bifida/meningomyelocele

84. Mild developmental delay

85. Enlarged Sylvian fissure

86. Cavum septum pellucidum

87. Pachygyria and polymicrogyria

88. Cortical dysgenesis or dysplasia

89. Arnold-Chiari anomaly

90. Upper airway obstruction in infancy

91. Absent or small adenoids, large palatine tonsils

92. Laryngeal web (anterior)

93. Large pharyngeal airway

94. Laryngomalacia

95. Arytenoid/corniculate hyperplasia

96. Pharyngeal hypotonia

97. Thin pharyngeal muscle

98. Asymmetric pharyngeal movement

99. Structurally asymmetric pharynx

100. Unilateral vocal cord paresis

101. Structurally asymmetric larynx

102. Reactive airway disease/asthma

103. Hypoplastic/aplastic kidney

104. Cystic kidneys

105. Inguinal hernias

106. Umbilical hernias

107. Diastasis recti

108. Diaphragmatic hernia

109. Malrotation of bowel

110. Hepatoblastoma and other tumors

111. Small hands and feet

112. Tapered digits

113. Short fingernails

114. Rough, red, scaly skin on hands and feet, morphea

115. Contractures

116. Triphalangeal thumbs

117. Polydactyly

118. Soft tissue syndactyly

119. Feeding difficulty

120. Failure to thrive

121. Chronic constipation

122. Gastroesophageal reflux (GER or GERD)

123. Nasal regurgitation

124. Irritability

125. Hypospadias

126. Cryptorchidism

127. Vesicoureteral reflux

128. Hydrocele

129. Scoliosis

130. Vertebral anomalies

131. Spina bifida occulta

132. Syrinx

133. Osteopenia

134. Sprengel anomaly

135. Talipes equinovarus and valgus deformity

136. Hypoplastic skeletal muscles

137. Hyperextensible/lax joints

138. Joint dislocations

139. Flat foot arches

140. Chronic leg pains

141. Extra ribs, rib fusion

142. Abundant scalp hair

143. Thin appearing skin (venous patterns easily visible)

144. Hypocalcemia

145. Hypoparathyroidism

146. Hypothyroidism/hyperthyroidism

147. Autoimmune thyroiditis

148. Hypoglycemia

149. Mild growth deficiency, relatively small stature (childhood)

150. Absent, hypoplastic thymus

151. Small pituitary gland (rare)

152. Immune deficiency or immune disorder

153. Velopharyngeal insufficiency (usually severe)

154. Severe hypernasality

155. Severe articulation impairment (glottal stops)

156. High pitched voice

157. Hoarseness

158. Language impairment (usually mild delay)

159. Learning disabilities

160. Concrete thinking, difficulty with abstraction and problem solving

161. Low IQ

162. Drop in IQ scores in school years

163. Attention deficit hyperactivity disorder (ADD/ADHD)

164. Autism spectrum disorder (ASD)

165. Schizophrenia

166. Bipolar disorder

167. Rapid or ultrarapid cycling of mood disorder

168. Mood disorder, dysthymia, cyclothymia

169. Depression

170. Hypomania

171. Manic depressive psychosis

172. Schizoaffective disorder

173. Impulsiveness

174. Flat affect

175. Social immaturity

176. Obsessive-compulsive disorder

177. Generalized anxiety disorder

178. Phobias

179. Severe startle response

180. Separation anxiety

181. Thrombocytopenia

182. Bernard-Soulier syndrome

183. Juvenile rheumatoid arthritis

184. Poor temperature regulation

185. Spontaneous oxygen desaturation without apnea

186. Vasomotor instability

187. Robin sequence

188. DiGeorge sequence

189. Potter sequence

190. Holoprosencephaly

# Index